Praise for *Breathe*

MW00586677

Dr. Shereen Lim has created a ground-breaking and absolutely necessary resource on a relatively unknown but ever-present epidemic affecting our children's breathing and sleep health. She presents an in-depth discussion on airway health – the diagnoses, treatment modalities, and outcomes for specific breathing problems – but more importantly, offers insight on underlying causes of clinical manifestations and how we can more proactively manage our kids' health, growth, and development. Dr. Lim's dental and sleep medicine expertise are evident in her careful explanations of the anatomic, behavioral, and functional factors related to sleep disorders, and I wholeheartedly believe that this book will shape the way we evaluate developmental sleep issues moving forward. If you are a new or experienced parent, a medical professional, or are in any way interested in population health, you owe it to yourself to read this book.

- **Audrey Yoon DDS MS**, *Pediatric Dentist and Orthodontist, Director of the Pacific Dental Sleep Medicine Fellowship and Co-Founding President of the World Dentofacial Sleep Medicine Society*

It is so exciting to finally have a science-based, patient friendly, comprehensive book covering airway health. Dr Lim does a magnificent job blending stories from her personal life, educational journey, and practice experience to make this an entertaining read. Our offices share a common goal of promoting airway health, optimal breathing, and restorative sleep. I plan to share *Breathe, Sleep, Thrive* with all my airway patients, highlighting the chapters that impact them and their family. Thank you, Shereen, for creating such a treasure. Your passion comes through in every page.

- **Jeff Rouse DDS**, *Private Practice Prosthodontist, San Antonio, Texas, USA Resident Faculty Spear Education*

Over the course of the last decade, Dr. Shereen Lim has travelled the world to study with experts and researchers in sleep and breathing from various disciplines, theories, backgrounds, and philosophies. *Breathe, Sleep, Thrive* is a beautifully written, easy to follow, highly up-to-date synopsis of the current best practices and research in our field. This book will be appreciated by patients, parents, and providers alike. I congratulate Dr. Lim on a job well done and thank her for her dedication in making airway health knowledge accessible to all.

- **Soroush Zaghi MD**, *Otolaryngologist- Sleep Surgeon, the Breathe Institute, Los Angeles*

Shereen has achieved in this book what many of us in the airway field aspire to do, that is in giving a big picture concept about the importance of sleep and breathing from womb to tomb. This is definitely not a book to refer to relevant chapters, but a must read from cover to cover so as to connect the dots in the big picture. She has hammered home the facts based on currently available research, some of it challenging traditional approaches which are still the accepted norm today. This book is not just for parents, but a must read for medical, dental and allied health practitioners especially those dealing with infants and children. It's a paradigm shift moving from traditional ethos to site specific, tailored and an integrated approach in dealing with this condition which is truly a global evolutionary pandemic.

- **Jeevanan Jahendran MS (ORL)**, *Otorhinolaryngologist, Pantai Hospital Kuala Lumpur*

Breathe, Sleep, Thrive is a comprehensive introduction to the important concept that early feeding, and breathing patterns can affect long term airway, teeth and jaw development. As a pediatric specialist that addresses airway and breathing problems in children down the line, it's very important for parents to be aware of these factors right from birth so that one can monitor and address these concerns before they become significant health issues. Parents should be aware that tongue ties can potentially cause feeding and breathing problems from infancy. This book is an invaluable resource to promote this awareness and address how one can prevent and or treat these conditions.

- **Umakanth Katwa MD**, *Medical Director of the Sleep Center for Pediatric Respiratory and Sleep Medicine at Boston Children's Hospital, Harvard Medical School*

Breathe, Sleep, Thrive will enable parents to lay the best foundation for their children's health. It guides parents about the patterns of jaw growth, mouth function, airway and breathing that facilitate the good sleep, essential for brain development and optimal daily functioning of infants and children. Dr Shereen Lim shares from her extensive experience and passion for airway health, backed by the research in a clear and easy to read manner. The book is also much needed for health practitioners to increase their knowledge in this new field where dentistry, orthodontics and medicine intersects with clinicians of different professions to promote and build better child health. I wish I had this book during my first parenting years. I will warmly recommend reading it to my patients, parents and colleagues.

- **Solveig Thorp Holmsen, MD, MPH**, *Senior Adviser Norwegian Institute of Public Health*

For several years, Dr. Shereen Lim set on a quest to explore something that she was never taught at dental school. The influence of airway and breathing on the general health of newborns infants, children, and adults. She travelled the world, visited many pioneers in the field and managed to accomplish a complete and full understanding with a very thorough clinical practice. Today, Shereen is one of the leading personas in this field and *Breathe, Sleep, Thrive* sheds light on a topic seldom taught or understood by most physicians, pediatricians and dentists. This book will definitely help parents grow a healthier generation.

- **Eyal Botzer DMD**, *Director of Pediatric Dentistry, Tel Aviv Medical Center, Israel*

I commend Dr. Lim for taking the complex topic of sleep abnormalities, craniofacial development and breathing physiology and analyzing the published evidence to demonstrate her contemporary management strategies. She perfectly synthesizes complex scientific principles with easy-to-read language that makes this book a must read for parents and medical professionals alike.

- **Bobby Ghaheri MD**, *Otolaryngologist, The Oregon Clinic, Portland*

Often the biggest barriers to truly life changing decisions is lack of even knowing what the choices are. If you've ever found yourself thinking, "If I only knew then what I know now" and you have (or soon will have) children, this book is for you. Dr. Shereen Lim has put together the information you need to pay attention to your child's breathing and what questions you should ask their health care providers. Armed with this in-depth preparation, you will have confidence to help your child achieve their best start in life.

- **Steve Carstensen DDS**, *Consultant to the American Dental Association (ADA) for Sleep Related Breathing Disorders, Chief Dental Editor of Dental Sleep Practice Magazine, and co-author of The Clinician's Handbook for Dental Sleep Medicine*

Dr. Shereen Lim dove down the rabbit hole of airway and sleep and became a passionate student, traveling around the world, learning from the best of the best to create a cutting-edge airway / sleep practice. In *Breathe, Sleep, Thrive* she has taken her academic knowledge and clinical experience to create an Airway Health guidebook for all parents and practitioners interested in helping children reach their full potential. It should be in every home of a parent or a future parent.

- **Howie Hindin DDS**, *Co-Founder and President of the American Academy of Physiological Medicine and Dentistry (AAPMD) and Founder of the Foundation for Airway Health*

The mouth is so important in providing almost all the necessary things our infants need to grow and develop. *Breathe, Sleep Thrive* is a well written, understandable source of information for new parents and offers them direction when things seem not to be what they feel they should be in their child's health. This book should be required reading not only for all parents of newborns, but all individuals involved in the care of infants.

- **Lawrence Kotlow DDS**, *Pediatric Dentist and author of SOS 4 TOTS: Tethered Oral Tissues, Tongue-Ties & Lip Ties*

In a world where sleep problems are endemic and regarded by many as 'normal in the trenches of parenting', we ask ourselves; 'does it have to be this way?' Sleep is a fundamental pillar of health that underpins every aspect of a child's development including executive brain function required for communication development that prepares children for life, and everything there-in. Delayed speech and language milestones may be one of the first markers parents or allied health professionals notice yet sleep screening is sadly not yet common practice. We could even say, our work as speech pathologists may be futile in the face of sleep wrecked kids and families and more poignantly true for sleep and breathing problems that may stem from poor facial development, that also impact speech! Kudos to Dr Lim In *'Breathe Sleep Thrive'* for outlining the critical role dentists and orthodontists may play in facilitating or restoring growth of oral structures that support healthy breathing during sleep with a 'fix before 6' philosophy, a book in which parents will find much wisdom.

- **Sharon Moore**, *Speech Pathologist, passionate Sleep Health Advocate, author of 'Sleep Wrecked Kids'*

Bestselling author and iconic entrepreneur Peter Thiel asks innovators this question in Zero to One: "What important truth do very few people agree with you on?" Dr. Shereen Lim's book effectively communicates her conviction in a key truth. Human health and well-being have their foundation in form and function, or anatomy and physiology. Optimizing form and function lies in interventions at key developmental milestones during a child's growth. Missed milestones may be restorable, but the results are often imperfect. As restoring airway health during sleep is a gateway to wellness, Dr. Lim takes us from zero to one, where her inspiration comes from the integration of form and function. When you are done with this book, you will join the ever-growing community that agrees with Dr. Lim. We were just in search of a perfect voice.

- **Stanley Liu MD**, *Sleep and Oral and Maxillofacial Surgeon, Associate Professor of Otolaryngology – Head and Neck Surgery and Director of the Stanford Sleep Surgery Fellowship, Stanford University School of Medicine*

BREATHE, SLEEP, THRIVE

Discover How Airway Health Can Unlock Your Child's Greater Health, Learning, and Potential

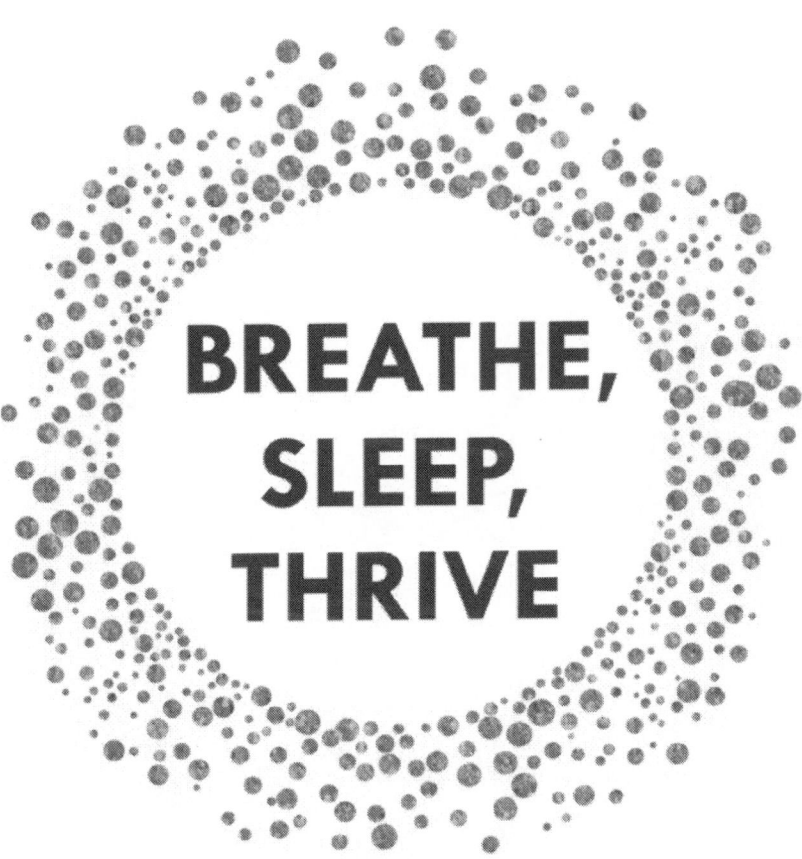

BREATHE, SLEEP, THRIVE

DR SHEREEN LIM

Breathe, Sleep, Thrive: Discover how airway health can unlock your child's greater health, learning, and potential

Cover Design by Aleksandar Milosavljevic Alek

ISBNs: 978-0-6455532-1-5 (paperback)
978-0-6455532-0-8 (eBook)

Published by Sparkle Publishing

Medical Advice Disclaimer

The information contained in the book Breathe, Sleep, Thrive, is provided for educational purposes only. It is not a substitute for professional medical advice, diagnosis, or treatment.

Always seek the advice of your physician or other qualified health care provider with any questions you may have regarding a medical condition or treatment and before using any information, idea, or products discussed.

While every effort has been made to ensure the accuracy of the information presented, neither the author nor the publisher assumes any responsibility for errors.

This book is dedicated to the countless people who have inspired and supported me to keep seeking better answers for patients, and to spread the message on airway health as wide as possible.

This includes the pioneers and researchers in the field, my mentors, friends and colleagues, partners in collaborative care, patients, parents, social media followers and those who have struggled to find answers with traditional health care silos.

It takes a village to create change in healthcare. Thank you for being a part of the shift towards airway health to ensure children can breathe, sleep, feed, grow and thrive to their fullest potential!

CONTENTS

INTRODUCTION

When you were planning to welcome your first child to the world, you may have read all the popular baby books or signed up for all the recommended classes to help you prepare. Informational sources like these strive to make you feel more equipped to handle parenthood for the first time.

However, when issues inevitably arise – such as tantrums, meltdowns, defiance, poor attention and concentration, hyperactivity, anxiety, difficulties with executive function and learning, speech and language concerns, and more – we realize that many important topics weren't included in our parent preparation manuals. Instead of recognizing these issues may all be symptoms of hidden breathing difficulties and fragmented, unrestorative sleep, we're running to the black hole of Dr Google and posting in Facebook groups to lament with other parents, normalizing problems that are quite significant. Soon, instead of recognizing that our initial concerns were valid, and a deeper root cause should be explored, we find comfort in the generalized philosophy that it shall pass someday.

The issue with this way of thinking is that many problems don't expire on their own, especially when they're related to proper breathing and sleeping. Instead, we accommodate their existence, or the problems shape into something else, compounding the initial cause that was never properly treated.

As parents, we aren't taught the telltale signs of our child's future health that can be seen as soon as the baby exits the womb, nor are we taught to observe the workings of their mouth as they grow. Dysfunctions of a child's mouth affect the way the jaw and airway structures grow and the way a child breathes. These are the earliest warning signs of potential sleep, cognitive, behavioral, and physical problems. They mean the muscles of the tongue and throat aren't working properly, which dominoes into other symptoms that continue to build on one another if left unaddressed. Most parents don't notice simply because we aren't sure what to look for.

Some of these early dysfunctions and warning signs include challenges with infant latching, swallowing of air and reflux-like symptoms, pacifier use, thumb-sucking, picky eating, over-reliance on soft processed diets, not chewing food properly, tongue thrusts, lisps and speech misarticulations, allergies and mouth breathing, and recurrent ear infections. These may sound like common situations, but this instinctual mindset further highlights the problem. We've simply become accustomed to them all – and the price we pay is our children's health.

Meltdowns are dismissed as normal child behaviour, with families walking on eggshells to manage them. Children are labelled and medicated with stimulants without anyone asking about their sleep. Even in less extreme cases, children may be falling short of their full potential. Schools require eyesight and hearing exams, but we are lacking a screening test to see how our children are breathing and sleeping – which is equally as crucial, especially on a learning front.

Many children with behavioural issues are diagnosed with ADHD based on subjective symptoms, often without anyone asking about their sleep. They are medicated with powerful stimulant medications with potentially serious side effects.

Crooked teeth are prevalent and a sign of poor structural development of the jaws. Braces are the go-to solution for many kids, but they only address the symptoms of a much bigger problem that is being avoided. Teeth are sometimes extracted to make space, with little regard to underlying poor jaw growth. Since the jaws are the bony support for our breathing passage, this represents a missed opportunity to optimize their airway and breathing.

And sadly, equally as related, we are witnessing a rise in obesity and other serious inflammatory diseases that were once considered adult problems in young children.

Whilst lifespans are increasing, more people are succumbing to degenerative diseases and reduced health-related quality of life into adulthood. An increasing proportion of the population is medicated from the cradle to the grave to manage diabetes, depression, high blood pressure, and other common illnesses and diseases.

Proper breathing is rarely discussed in parenting guides, yet it's the most important function as a baby enters the world, even more important than food and water. It's the one thing we absolutely cannot live without. The way we breathe will impact every aspect of our health, learning, growth, and future health – so why is it not talked about in a way that will help us prepare for all the warning signs of compromised airway health?

In modern societies, jaws are shrinking (more on this in Chapter 2), causing difficulties in sleep and breathing, but preventative measures are rarely discussed. Breathing difficulties during sleep are linked to unrestorative sleep, enhanced stress, inflammation, and oxygen deprivation, which means increased risk of virtually every chronic inflammatory disease.

Many people are unaware that there's an epidemic of breathing difficulties unfolding before our very eyes. I don't share this to alarm you; this is a call for a reformed approach to growth and development. Let's not watch and wait when symptoms arise, only moving to treat extremes. We don't need to wait for our children to develop snoring or obstructive sleep apnoea or crooked teeth; we can take preventative action.

We become better advocates for the health of our kids (and ourselves) when we have a thorough understanding of airway health, a topic that's not discussed as often as it should be.

If you have indeed experienced any of the above symptoms or know children in your life who have, you'll want to learn more about airway health. Noticing warning signs early allows you to take the right course of action and set your child up for a healthy life as soon as possible. A bonus is that doing so will also alleviate the pain you're experiencing as a parent, because healthy children equate to happy families. No one has to suffer. There is a better way – and it starts with being proactive in your child's health, not reactive as modern society has trained us to be.

The great news is that we are at the start of a new era of growing recognition of these hidden airway problems and their developmental origins. We now know there is a lot we can do to optimize sleep and breathing and significantly alter the lifetime trajectory of problems early in childhood. There is also a growing number of healthcare professionals from different disciplines (such as lactation consultants, speech and feeding therapists, dental professionals, Ear Nose and Throat specialists or ENTs, occupational therapists, and many more) on the same page, working to help minimize these problems from birth.

I was one of Australia's first dentists to obtain a qualification in the dental management of adult snoring and obstructive sleep apnoea. Time after time, I witnessed adult patients struggling and falling short of their full potential with low energy, brain fog, depression, and worsening related health conditions. Many people fail to realize that the onset of most adult health problems – including breathing dysfunction – begins when you're born. The way the mouth and throat muscles work in-utero and during infancy, and the way the jaws grow in the earliest years of life influence the structure and function of our airway into adulthood, determining how collapsible our airways will be during sleep and our risk of breathing difficulties. I could see the signs of poor mouth development and function in my adult patients and realized the many missed opportunities for intervention that could have made their breathing easier.

The foundation of our health is set in the first few years of life, which is why we need to intervene early at the first sign of an issue, and my passion for this is the reason my practice has shifted to early intervention to optimize mouth function, jaw and airway development, breathing, and sleep for children. The biggest key to optimal health and wellness and unlocking their highest potential is to develop and promote proper nasal breathing.

Breathe, Sleep, Thrive will help parents who want to understand hidden airway problems from childhood to adulthood and what they can do about them. Your child may have sleep and breathing issues and, if so, you know they are not rising to their full potential. Or maybe you want to know how to tell your child is on track and if there are things you can do to optimize their sleep and breathing. Some of you may even be facing problems yourself, which has made you more driven to avoid your child facing the same challenges. By the end of this book, you'll be so empowered by airway health knowledge that you'll know exactly what signs to look for and the steps to take to confidently set your child up for a lifetime of better health.

Part I highlights the importance of good sleep during early childhood, and will help you recognise breathing problems, the impact, and signs and symptoms to be aware of. You will begin to discover the growing epidemic of airway disorders affecting our sleep and physical, mental, and emotional health which are robbing us of our full potential. I will help you begin to recognise the underlying airway problems to create a shift away from managing symptoms and disease, to a focus on airway health.

Part II is about the different airway developmental milestones – from infant feeding to choosing orthodontic treatment to address your child's crooked teeth. You will gain a better appreciation for the key building blocks for optimal breathing, mouth function, and stimulation of proper jaw and airway development, and the different choices to promote a better path that can be made as children grow.

Part III is about screening and identifying children at risk of problems, and the various paths that can help their breathing and airway development get back on track when key oral milestones have been missed. I will conclude with a chapter on adult airway health, including newer options that can restore good airway structure and function for adults. In contrast to traditional approaches to manage symptoms, I want to ensure every person has the choice to restore airway health and nasal breathing to unlock their greatest health and wellness.

Read this book either cover to cover or look at the contents and skip straight to the relevant chapter if you have specific concerns about your child's development. You may start connecting the dots between seemingly unrelated issues your child is facing. The common thread will be some sort of oral dysfunction, such as abnormal sucking, feeding, or swallowing, or mouth breathing originating early in life, which leads to poor jaw and airway development as a catalyst for many disorders and diagnoses.

One of the challenges we face in the airway health awareness movement is the compartmentalization of healthcare. Quite often, health professionals may be true experts in their field, but they do not necessarily see the big picture of how everything interconnects, and they may not be familiar with the latest evidence of how the mouth and sleep are linked. It may be hard to find readily available information with practitioners in your area until there is greater emphasis on sleep and breathing and new research is disseminated more widely through educational institutions. With both dental and sleep medicine backgrounds, and the opportunity to care for the spectrum of patients, from infants to adults with end stage breathing problems, I will integrate the spectrum of information for you. My mission is to highlight the path of addressing root causes rather than managing symptoms. I want more children growing up breathing and sleeping easier, and thriving, to prevent the problems that I have seen in my adult patients.

I hope this book will help you find more answers for your child. I hope it will empower you to ask more questions, seek alternative options, and know that the choices you make for your child are informed.

Mostly, I hope this book provides you with exactly the information you need to lean into the significance of airway health and become part of the movement to change lives – both now and in the future.

PART I

SLEEP AND AIRWAY HEALTH

1

SLEEP AND BREATHING

Sleep is a key pillar of health. It is vital for our immune systems and helps us stay healthier and safer, learn better, and be more productive.

The need for sleep is particularly important in the first three years of life. In the first year of life, the brain size doubles and at the end of three years, it has attained 80% of its adult volume.[1] During this time, maximal synapses – or connections – in the brain are forming, a process which wires the brain, forming the foundations for learning and memory.

Another significant aspect of brain development is the maturation of the prefrontal cortex, otherwise known as the brain's control centre. It is involved in executive function, or the higher-level skills and processes involved in achieving goals, mental control, and self-regulation. This area is also important for short-term or working memory, speech production, and language and brain development peaks around puberty.

Many books on sleep focus on good routines, sleep associations, and normal sleep times by age.

But quality is as important as quantity. Airway problems and difficulty breathing are commonly overlooked causes of disturbed sleep in children. They don't allow children to enter the deep phases of sleep that are required for restoration, attention and concentration, and daytime function. In some cases, airway problems can also result in mini episodes of oxygen deprivation, chronic stress, and increased risk of health problems down the road.

When I first ask parents for their impressions of their child's sleep, a common response is, "My child's a great sleeper, once they are down, they don't wake up." It doesn't occur to check how they are breathing through the night – especially the latter half of the night, when children experience the deepest sleep and are most vulnerable to airway problems.

The problem is that parents don't always know the signs and symptoms of disturbed breathing they should look for.

This means key warning signs like tossing and turning, snoring, teeth grinding, or mouth breathing are being missed, and therefore children remain untreated and vulnerable to chronic deprivation of restorative sleep.

> **A sleeping child should be quiet, still, and breathing through their nose with their mouth closed.**

Whilst some parents may think their child's snore is adorable, it really should be concerning. It's a sign that there is restriction of airflow and that there may be increasing breathing difficulties down the track. It doesn't necessarily have to be as loud as dad's snoring. Any sound is an indication of resistance to airflow.

Snoring is also the most common symptom of a condition called Obstructive Sleep Apnoea (OSA), which is characterized by collapses of the throat that last for ten seconds or more during sleep, despite the brain's normal signals to the muscles to breathe. The structural narrowing of the airway leads to arousals from sleep and oxygen deprivation. OSA affects 5% of children. It is as common as asthma, which is typically regarded as the most common childhood disease. The problem with OSA is that it's harder to notice, and a lot of children remain untreated and at risk of serious consequences.[2]

If someone were choking your child during sleep, I'm sure you would be livid. Children with OSA have brief episodes of suffocation on their own, all night long, night after night.

These are the signs and symptoms to be aware of:

- open mouth breathing
- audible breathing, snoring, or gasping
- restlessness, tossing, and turning
- unusual sleep positions – neck hyperextension, stomach sleeping, bum in the air
- sweating
- teeth grinding
- bedwetting
- frequent or unexplained awakenings
- night terrors
- unrefreshed on waking
- tired or wired through the day
- poor concentration and attention
- concerns with behaviour, emotional regulation, anxiety
- concerns with learning, school performance

Mounting research links obstructive sleep breathing (including snoring) with wide-ranging consequences:

- high blood pressure and other cardiovascular problems
- metabolic disease
- poor growth – related to reduced growth hormone which is secreted in deep sleep
- increased risk of neurocognitive and behavioural problems
- speech and language concerns
- bedwetting
- poor facial development

Approximately half of children with OSA will be obese and overweight. These children are more likely to have the most severe breathing disturbances, metabolic disorders, insulin resistance, and cardiovascular and high blood pressure.

Even children who are not obese but have OSA show elevated markers that could predict future disease. For example, new research shows children with obstructive breathing have increased chemical messengers that promote plaque build ups in the arteries, amplifying the risk of strokes and heart disease.[3]

In general, for the non-obese child without any medical syndromes, the most immediate problem will be what happens to the brain and learning potential.[4]

There are two main mechanisms behind these problems.

The first is that these breathing difficulties lead to fragmented sleep. To imagine this, think about being woken up by a phone ringing multiple times per hour and only getting sleep between each call. Your sleep would not only be broken up but would fail to progress into the deepest levels. Even as an adult, we're not going to feel great in the morning or perform at our best. But what if that was happening every single night?

As a result of this fragmentation, snoring even without oxygen deprivation is linked to unrestorative sleep and reduced attention and concentration.[5,6] These children may be distractible or even disruptive in class and their learning will be affected. Unlike adults who become tired or lethargic, a sleep deprived child may present with symptoms of overtiredness. They may become wired, fidgety, be constantly moving to keep themselves awake, or have poor emotional regulation and be prone to meltdowns and tantrums or defiance. Rather than assume these behaviours are a normal part of childhood or the "terrible twos," it's important to rule out airway issues and unrestorative sleep.

When children present with symptoms like lack of attention, hyperactivity, and impulsive behaviour, they can sometimes be diagnosed with ADHD. If we don't first rule out airway problems, the problem of side effects with stimulant medications is compounded by the fact that we're giving children the opposite of what they really need – a good night's sleep. There are numerous studies which have demonstrated an improvement in ADHD symptoms in children who had a restricted airway addressed through removing enlarged adenoids and tonsils in the throat.[7,8]

It is essential to pay attention to breathing difficulties as soon as they appear. Even if breathing difficulties from the first year of life resolve, the risk of behavioural and socio-emotional problems including inattention/hyperactivity, anxiety and depression, peer problems, aggressiveness, and rule breaking in later childhood may still be increased.

In a landmark study following up 11,000 children by Bonuck and coworkers, children who had a history of mouth breathing, snoring, and gasping during sleep from as young as six months were more likely to have these behavioural and socio-emotional issues by age four to seven years.[9] Bonuck's research focused on five behavioural domains including: inattention/hyperactivity, emotional symptoms (anxiety and depression), peer problems, conduct problems (aggressiveness and rule-breaking), and prosocial behavior (sharing, helpfulness, etc.).

The most affected domain was inattention/hyperactivity, and the most affected children were those who had symptoms peak at age 30 months and reduce after. This study supports the fact that the early years of life are a critical period of development where mouth breathing, snoring, and OSA are particularly detrimental and may have a degree of irreversibility.

Based on this and other evidence, the American Academy of Pediatrics endorsed the guideline that children should be screened for mouth breathing, snoring, or gasping during sleep from the first year of life.[10] The unfortunate reality is that this is often overlooked in clinical practice.

The second detrimental impact on the brain is the loss of grey matter. Grey matter is the outermost layer of the brain that is involved in higher processing of sensory information, memory and cognitive function, control of movement, and emotions. One of the most compelling studies examined over 10,000 children enrolled in the Adolescent Brain Cognitive Development (ABCD) study who had MRI scans of their brain.[11] They found that children who snored or gasped during sleep had smaller volumes of grey matter in their frontal lobes.

These structural changes in the brain may be the beginnings of the changes that are now linked to obstructive sleep breathing and the memory loss seen in dementia and Alzheimer's in adults. What if treating this condition in childhood could help stave off the second leading cause of death in Australia, and a despairing problem for which there is no cure or treatment for?

Neurocognitive deficits are thought to be a result of the interplay between inattention and grey matter loss in critical areas of the brain.

Menzie and co-workers from Sydney conducted a systematic review that pooled the results of 63 studies to analyze the relationship between disturbed breathing during sleep, and objective measures of neurocognitive function.[12] They published their results in the journal Sleep Medicine Reviews in 2022. They found breathing disturbances from snoring to obstructive sleep apnoea were linked to deficits across all aspects of neurocognitive function including:

- intelligence
- attention/executive function
- memory
- language
- visual spatial skills

Overall, children with primary snoring (without oxygen deprivation) had comparable and sometimes higher levels of deficits than those children who had obstructive sleep apnoea. This finding was attributed to the disturbance in sleep from increased fragmentation and arousals in primary snorers.

One of the very first studies to link abnormal sleep breathing with a negative impact on academic performance was by Dr David Gozal and team., published in Paediatrics in 1998.[13] They found an increase of obstructive sleep breathing amongst first graders who were in the lowest 10th percentile of their class in school performance. The children who had removal of their adenoids and tonsils saw improvements in their academics in subsequent years compared to those who went without treatment.

A later study by that same team found that children with lower academic performance in middle school were more likely to have snored during early childhood.[14] This first suggested some degree of the neurocognitive deficit may be irreversible – and that a learning debt may develop with obstructive breathing early in life – hampering subsequent school performance. It's sort of like replenishing water in a leaky bucket.

Oxygen deprivation subjects children to a decrease of eight IQ points on average, and although this may never become apparent, for example, in a child with a high IQ of 180, a child with an average IQ of 100 could see their success later in life affected negatively.[15]

Sleep-disturbed breathing often does not receive the attention it deserves from mainstream healthcare because of the lack of professional training in sleep medicine. Many physicians have yet to understand the seriousness of snoring and therefore the effects. Dr David Gozal underscores the seriousness of sleep-disturbed breathing: "The quality of life of a child that has sleep apnoea is equivalent to that of a child with cancer receiving chemotherapy".[16] The difference here is that we would recognise the impact of the cancer and understand the child's suffering but snoring and sleep apnoea often go unnoticed despite what they're doing to our children.

> The key takeaways, and what I hope that you will help spread word on, are "Don't Ignore The Snore," and if your child is diagnosed with ADHD, make sure you have ruled out airway problems prior to medicating.

Remember, children don't grow out of these issues – they grow into them. They end up falling short of their full potential and we don't really know who they would have become if they hadn't been affected.

Traditionally, there has been a one-size-fits-all approach to managing this problem.

The most-studied intervention, which is proven to significantly alleviate symptoms of breathing difficulties, is surgical removal of enlarged adenoids and tonsils, or masses of immune tissue that are crowding the throat.

But multi-centre research tells us that up to 80% of children will still have a significant degree of breathing dysfunction after surgery.[17] In addition, research tells us that many children who are seemingly "cured" will have a recurrence of symptoms when they are older.[18,19] I know this to be the case because a great bulk of my work is addressing concerns with persistent mouth breathing, snoring, and teeth grinding for children who have had this surgery.

> My aim is to help you better understand that this is a multifactorial problem, and as such will require an integrative team approach that involves dental professionals, ENT surgeons, speech pathologists, and more to precisely address each child's unique risk factors and ensure nasal breathing.

It can also help us to be proactive and intervene early. In the next chapter, I will take you deeper into the many factors that make up airway health (including the importance of nasal breathing, proper tongue mobility and function, and good jaw development) to empower you to advocate for your child's health.

2

AIRWAY HEALTH

My involvement in sleep medicine, managing snoring and obstructive sleep apnoea, began with adult patients.

My interest was prompted out of frustration with my husband's snoring. It was disturbing my sleep, and I was somewhat aware that dental appliances were an effective option to help manage this. One night, when my patience finally ran out, I jumped out of bed and began googling and learning about dental devices for snoring. This led me to my decision: I was going to learn more and become qualified – not only to manage my husband, but also to fill a void for other spouses in the same boat!

I soon learned that snoring was not just a noisy annoyance in the bedroom. The repetitive threat to normal air intake associated with snoring could result in unrestorative sleep, oxygen deprivation, chronic stress, and inflammation, all of which could create havoc with people's energy, mood, health, and daily function.

It was despairing to see how many of my patients were struggling and living short of their potential. Some were juggling multiple medications and chronic health conditions, or suffering from anxiety, depression, headaches, brain fog, and constant tiredness or fatigue, but nobody had asked them about their sleep or breathing. I could start to see and recognise that if we knew the right questions to ask and what to look for, there were early warning signs (and many of them in the mouth) that could be identified long before the disturbed sleep became apparent. We were missing the opportunity to set up a better path of breathing for children, so they didn't grow into adults with big problems. I'm passionate about helping more people recognise the signs and create a shift from treating disease and symptoms to addressing root causes and promoting airway health and optimal breathing from infancy.

This is why I now largely focus on children. Being involved in an integrative approach to managing airway problems in children is rewarding because it not only helps them live up to their full potential, but it can change an entire family dynamic. When children sleep well, so do their parents. When children are well rested and have less struggles with behaviour and learning, their parents can be more present, enjoy them, and return attention to the rest of the family.

The approach to airway health is slowly reaching a tipping point, and rightly so. Breathing is vital for life. It's more important than diet or exercise, and the way we breathe deserves as much attention, if not more, as there is on physical, heart, brain, mental, or gut health.

Airway health is about optimal breathing around the clock. "Optimal" means unrestricted nasal breathing day and night. It also means paying attention to good jaw and airway development and ensuring the proper function of the tongue and other throat muscles that form our upper airway from birth. When we breathe well, we sleep, grow, learn, and live well.

I'm going to highlight some of the pitfalls of modern healthcare and sleep medicine while also exploring what we need to pay attention to as an alternative approach to airway health.

Snoring and OSA are part of a spectrum of increasing breathing difficulties collectively described as obstructive Sleep Disturbed Breathing. It's important to understand that these problems are a symptom of narrow and restricted airways and poor breathing both day and night. There is no gene for snoring. These issues have their developmental origins early in life.

The underlying poor airway structure can result from a combination of the following:

- excess soft tissue inside the nose and throat such as swelling from allergies and other inflammation, and enlarged adenoids and tonsils
- narrow or receded jaws that form the floor of the nose, space for the tongue and structural support of the upper airway
- the tone of the muscles that keep the upper airway open. Poor muscle patterns include open mouth and low tongue posture.

During the day, these structural deficiencies may not necessarily pose a problem. But at night, when the throat muscles are more relaxed, the reflexes that keep the upper airway open are not as active, and the tissues of the soft palate and tongue are more likely to fall back into our throats when we are lying on our backs. The net results are increased airway collapsibility and compromise to the smooth passage of airflow into the lungs.

In other words, these problems are not exactly "sleep breathing" problems but are, in a more accurate sense, airway problems that predispose people to more difficulties during sleep.

SPECTRUM OF OBSTRUCTIVE SLEEP DISTURBED BREATHING (oSDB)

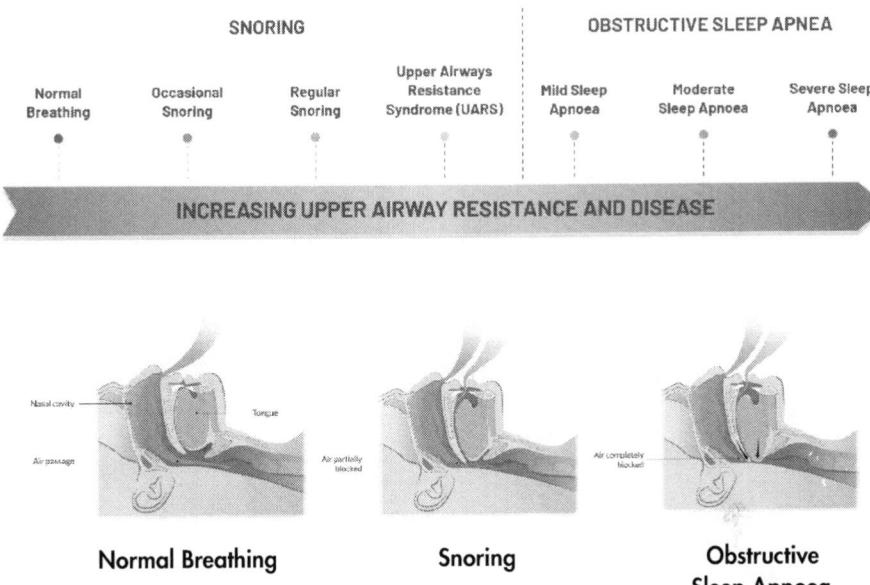

SNORING

OBSTRUCTIVE SLEEP APNEA

| Normal Breathing | Occasional Snoring | Regular Snoring | Upper Airways Resistance Syndrome (UARS) | Mild Sleep Apnoea | Moderate Sleep Apnoea | Severe Sleep Apnoea |

INCREASING UPPER AIRWAY RESISTANCE AND DISEASE

Nasal cavity
Tongue
Air passage

Air partially blocked

Air completely blocked

Normal Breathing

Snoring

Obstructive Sleep Apnoea

At the most severe end of the spectrum we have Obstructive Sleep Apnoea (OSA), characterised by prolonged collapses of the airway despite efforts to breathe. The main measure used to define the severity of OSA is the Apnoea–Hypopnea Index (AHI). This represents the total number of breathing stoppages (apnoeas) and periods of airway restriction and reduced airflow (hypopneas) lasting more than 10 seconds each per hour of sleep. 'These events are counted when they result in a brief awakening or arousal from sleep, or reduced oxygenation in the blood. The severity is classified as shown in the following table:

	Adults	**Children**
Mild	5 to 15 events	1 to 5 events
Moderate	15 to 30 events	5 to 10 events
Severe	30 or more	More than 10 events

Compared to adults who require five or more of these prolonged events to occur per hour of sleep for a diagnosis of OSA, children have a reduced threshold of one episode per hour, as their developing brains are highly susceptible to oxygen deprivation.

Often, a person will have no recollection these episodes of mini-suffocation are occurring. They may simply feel unrefreshed on waking, have unexplained tiredness or mood disorder, or excessive daytime sleepiness. Children may present more "wired" than tired. Over time, this breathing abnormality is linked to chronic stress and inflammation and impacts virtually every system in the body. In fact, it would be hard to name a chronic health condition that does not have a direct or indirect link to OSA.

You now know OSA is linked to increased risk of behavioural and learning problems in children. In adults, it is linked to increased risk of wide-ranging consequences depicted below.

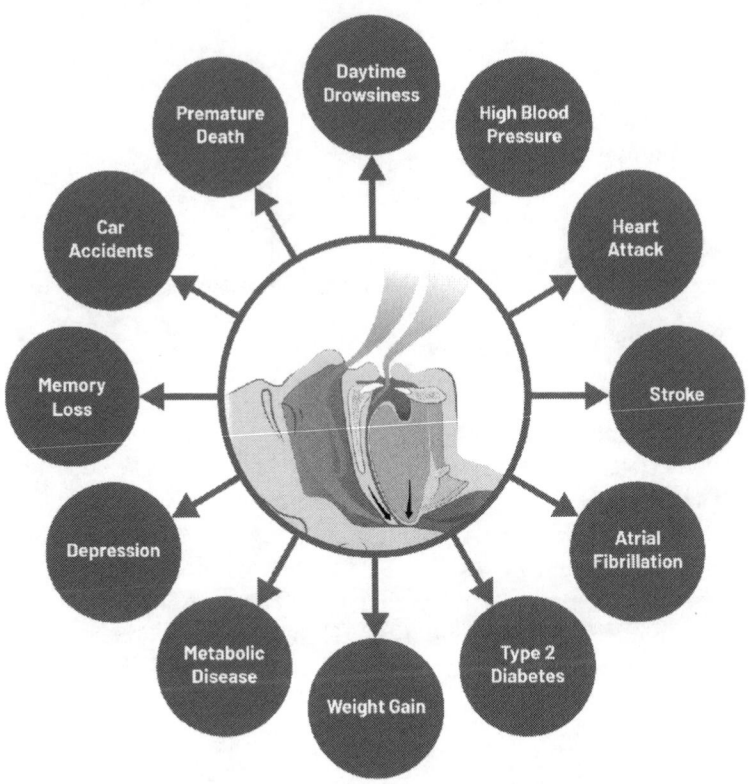

It's been estimated that up to 85% of people with OSA have not been diagnosed. The problem is that we manage many of the symptoms above by taking medications. Health care is compartmentalised, and people see multiple specialists for various conditions, which are treated individually. The common contribution of poor airway health and unrestorative sleep is overlooked.

In the last chapter, I discussed how children could be misdiagnosed with ADHD and medicated without addressing underlying airway problems. A parallel situation in adults is the misdiagnosis of clinical depression.

In a Perth study by Dr Cass Edwards and team published in 2015 in the Journal of Clinical Sleep Medicine, 73% of 293 patients diagnosed with sleep apnoea had depressive symptoms. After treatment of their OSA with CPAP (continuous positive airway pressure), only 4% had any clinically significant depression.[1] Of the 41 patients who were treated that had originally reported feelings of self-harm or the perception that they were 'better off dead', none of them had persisting suicidal thoughts at a three-month follow up. Dr Edwards is a friend and a lifesaver, literally, helping people on the brink of despair through her work on sleep education - giving them answers and hope that allows them to turn their lives around.

Did you know that 30-50% of people with hypertension have OSA, and this increases to up to 85% in those patients who have refractory hypertension, or whose blood pressure is not controlled with the use of three medications?[2]

But that's just the tip of the iceberg. OSA is the most extreme form (or end stage problem) of Sleep Disturbed Breathing. If we focus too much on this, we are missing the subtle pre-cursor forms that are more likely to occur in populations such as children, thin individuals, and pre-menopausal women. They may not be as prone to prolonged collapses of the airway and oxygen deprivation, but these groups are still vulnerable to airflow restriction and the consequences of fragmented sleep.

For example, in **Upper Airways Resistance Syndrome (UARS)**, the sympathetic nervous system is on high alert to defend against the constant threat to adequate oxygenation throughout the night. It sends a signal to increase efforts to breathe to compensate and maintain airflow. Despite there being no complete collapses of the airway and drops in oxygen, the body is in a state of chronic stress or "fight or flight." It's like getting prodded or having an alarm clock go off repeatedly throughout the night. These constant arousals fragment sleep, and the body does not enter the deep, restorative phases. Adults may present with unexplained tiredness or fatigue, while children may be lethargic or display symptoms of overtiredness or hyperactivity.

UARS is associated with the chronic dumping of stress hormones in the body. As a result, teeth grinding, tension headaches, anxiety, insomnia, or irritable bowel syndrome (IBS) type symptoms and other "rest and digest" dysfunctions may occur. Sadly, for some, it is their normal and they have no idea they are falling short. UARS may be accompanied by anxiety that is assumed to be psychological when it may be a physiological response to the chronic stress of airway/breathing restriction. Have you recognised these symptoms in your child? If so, this may be an area worth exploring.

This pattern of increased breathing effort is thought to be more prevalent than OSA, yet UARS is not as well recognised or studied. It is often overlooked in children who have symptoms of poor sleep and daytime function but have a negative sleep study result for OSA. In sleep medicine, we need to stop focusing on the very arbitrary ten second airway blockages and better recognise and manage UARS too. The emphasis sleep medicine places on numbers is deceiving; if someone's airway is only blocked for nine seconds instead of ten, does this mean they are fine, or does it mean that our current system and methods of diagnosis are in desperate need of an overhaul? I will mention this in a later chapter – but the late Dr Christian Guilleminault who developed the AHI expressed regret about this later in his career. He spent his final years highlighting the need for more attention to airflow limitation without the drops in oxygenation, especially for children.[3]

Snoring is the most well-recognised symptom of breathing abnormalities, and its first onset can be a warning sign of increasing difficulties with airflow down the track. Snoring fragments sleep and robs it of its restorative benefits.

> **Snoring fragments sleep and robs it of its restorative benefits.**

The so-called "primary snoring" (snoring without any reductions in oxygenation) is linked to grey matter losses and increased risks of behavioural problems in children. In adults, snoring is an independent risk factor for stroke[4] – the third biggest cause of death in Australia. The vibrations can dislodge a clot that forms in the arterial plaque of the carotid artery in the neck. When this passes to the brain and blocks a vessel, it can interrupt blood flow to the brain. This is one of the most common ways a stroke can occur.

Although more people are catching on that snoring is a warning sign or problems, I want parents to be aware that mouth breathing is an even earlier warning sign they need to look out for, which I will discuss more in Chapter 3.

In the meantime, here's an easy motto you can share with your kids: **The nose is for breathing, and the mouth is for chewing and speaking.** This sounds simple but is often overlooked and needs to be emphasised.

After managing many children and adults with sleep breathing disorders (and their wide-ranging consequences), I'm calling for a change in sleep medicine.

> **We must focus more on good breathing and sleep as a key pillar of health rather than focusing solely on treating disease and managing symptoms with medications and surgery.**

Let's focus less on the extreme dysfunction that occurs in OSA, and more on promoting airway health and nasal breathing.

Let's recognise the subtle precursor forms as opportunities for intervention, and let's do what we can to reinforce or secure nasal breathing for children from as young as infancy.

The other big shifts I'm calling for are greater integration in healthcare and a change in the way that we view crooked teeth. This is largely a symptom of poor jaw development, and this means sub-optimal breathing.

I mentioned earlier that all these airway and sleep breathing difficulties have a component of the structural narrowing of the airway.

Many health care professionals recognise the problems that narrow the inside of the airway – like enlarged adenoids and tonsils, floppy soft palates, deviated septums, and swelling or inflammation that comes from allergies, obesity, or reflux disease. But equally important is the outer frame of the airway, which is determined by the jaws. Good jaw development in childhood is another key to a lifetime of optimal airway health.

The upper jaw forms the nasal floor and has a huge influence on nasal cross section and airflow in the nasal passages. It also forms the housing for the tongue. Both jaws offer the rigid structural support for the collapsible tube of airway muscles in our throat.

Underdeveloped jaws that are narrowed or recessed are a well-established risk factor in the development of obstructive breathing in infants through adults. This is why some of the most effective treatment options for managing these breathing problems involve addressing deficient jaw structures. These include palate or upper jaw widening, utilizing devices that reposition the lower jaw forward during sleep, and double jaw advancement surgery.

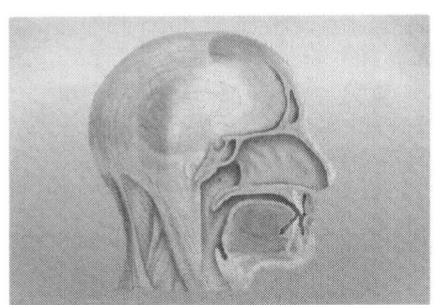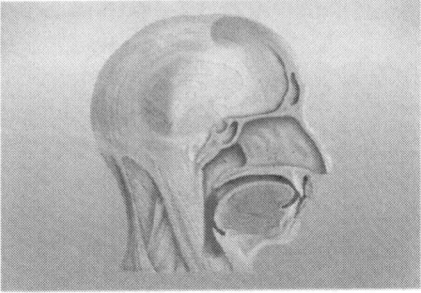

Shared and used with permission by James Nestor, Breath: The New Science of a Lost Art.

The wider and more forward the jaws are, the more space for the tongue to be housed properly and out of the airway. You can also see in the left image above there is more space for the airway behind them, and it also offers greater support or tension for the collapsible tube of throat or upper airway muscles. This allows air to pass more freely and reduces the collapsibility of the airway during sleep.

When the upper jaw and the nasal passages are narrow and the jaws are not properly positioned forward in the face, the airway becomes pinched. It takes more effort to breathe air through a smaller pipe. This can be likened to sucking hard on a straw. The airway then becomes more susceptible to collapsing or obstructing with every breath in.

Holistic dentist Dr Felix Liao describes the condition of underdeveloped jaws as "impaired mouth syndrome" in his book *Six Foot Tiger, Three-Foot Cage*.[5] This analogy describes the stress created from a mouth that is too small to house the tongue. The tongue is forced into the airway where it becomes a caged tiger, causing chronic oxygen and sleep deprivation, as well as various other symptoms throughout the body – like teeth grinding and high blood pressure.

By the time we address these problems in adulthood, we are relying on band-aid solutions like CPAP or dental appliances which do not resolve the problem (and which a patient is reliant on for life), or more invasive jaw surgeries. Quite often these adults are the same children who have struggled with breathing difficulties and symptoms like ADHD, difficulties learning, and bedwetting since childhood.

There is growing professional awareness that we need to optimise the jaws early to optimize sleep, breathing, and learning potential, and to prevent the development of obstructive breathing and the increased risks of physical, mental, and emotional problems that come along with it. But things are still moving slowly, and if we wait too long for new research and thinking to be widely disseminated, we are going to be missing the boat for many children.

Having crooked teeth is the most obvious first sign of poor jaw development, and yet it is common practice for orthodontists to watchfully wait and do nothing until around the age of 12. This coincides with when the permanent teeth come through and 90% of jaw development is complete. The rationale is that achieving straight teeth at this later stage is more efficient, with less burnout for the child and family. Sometimes this is done even at the expense of healthy permanent teeth that need to be removed to alleviate dental crowding. We miss the opportunity to modify jaw development to build a better foundation for the teeth to fit whilst a child is growing most rapidly. But even more importantly, we are missing the boat to get the skeletal support for the airway growing the right way so we can breathe best for life. If this is not being incorporated in orthodontic curriculums, then many children are being seen on a regular "watch and wait" basis whilst problems worsen, without them ever being asked about their breathing and sleep. This is changing more so in the US, but until this change happens locally, you need to be able to advocate for your child when there are problems.

During my dental sleep medicine course, I learned of research by sleep medicine pioneer Dr Christian Guilleminault demonstrating that widening the palate could improve breathing and reduce Obstructive Sleep Apnoea in children. Widening the palate and making more room for the teeth had always made sense to me and knowing it could improve breathing made me determined not to have to go down the path of extracting teeth for my own children.

I decided I was going to learn more about interceptive orthodontics and palate expansion, so I started my venture into orthodontics with a two-year mini residency in Dentofacial Orthopaedics and Orthodontics with world renowned orthodontist Dr Derek Mahony from Sydney.

At that time in 2014, I was at a paediatric sleep medicine conference where I had the chance to first meet Dr Guilleminault. I told him that his work had inspired me to learn and offer palate expansion, to which he replied, "if you are looking at doing palate expansion, you are too late!" At the time, I was surprised and had no idea what he meant. That moment was a spark that ignited my desire to keep learning and finding out more about the root causes of poor jaw and airway development.

The traditional age for early interceptive orthodontics is age seven to eight years. The Australian Society of Orthodontists recommends a child should have their first orthodontic evaluation by age seven to eight years. The flaw with that is that the jaws are growing most rapidly in the earliest years of life. In fact, 60% of the adult sized face is attained by the age of six years. We need to address the root causes of poor jaw development in the first years of life in order to get our children on the track to optimal breathing sooner.

As dentists, we have been effective in promoting the prevention of dental diseases such as decay and gum disease, but there has been very little focus on understanding origins of crooked teeth and how we can intervene to minimize the problem.

One argument is that poor facial and jaw development is purely genetic, and that we must resign ourselves to it being beyond our control. However, dental anthropologists have found that shrinking jaws, crooked teeth, and impacted wisdom teeth are a relatively new phenomenon, and therefore cannot be genetic or related to a change in our DNA code.

Instead, shrinking jaws and crooked teeth are thought to be an epigenetic phenomenon[6] – that is, modern lifestyles are impacting the way our genes are expressed. Whether it be changes in diet, infant feeding preferences, pacifiers, or an increasing prevalence of mouth breathing, the way our muscles work determines how our jaws grow.

CROOKED TEETH AND CHANGES IN DIET CONSISTENCY

The skulls of hunters and gatherers had forward-projecting jaws, broad mouths, expansive sinuses, and nasal passages, and plenty of room for their tongue and airway. They fed on game, wild roots, and vegetables and had to chew intensely to extract their nutrients.

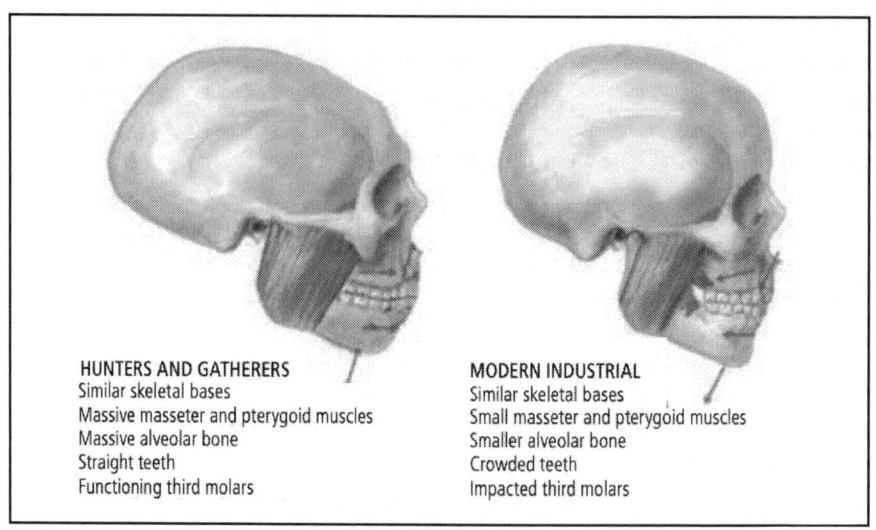

HUNTERS AND GATHERERS
Similar skeletal bases
Massive masseter and pterygoid muscles
Massive alveolar bone
Straight teeth
Functioning third molars

MODERN INDUSTRIAL
Similar skeletal bases
Small masseter and pterygoid muscles
Smaller alveolar bone
Crowded teeth
Impacted third molars

Image used with permission by Drs Jerry Rose and Richard Roblee, with credit to Carlson and Van Gerven 1977 for original image and concept

Dental crowding was first apparent around 10,000 years ago, coinciding with the agricultural revolution and the transition from foraging to farming. There was an introduction of tools and cooking which pulverized food and made it less tough. With less chewing, there was a dramatic reduction in the size of the jaw bones. Overall, with the transition from active hunting and gathering, there was less need for robust skeletal support.

However, it wasn't until approximately 300 to 400 years ago with the Industrial Revolution that crooked teeth became more widely prevalent. At this time there was a major shift from fresh, raw, and natural foods to canned, highly processed foods and tenderised meats. This includes burgers, stews, soups, and breads. Overall, there was a reduction in the spectrum of nutrients and a simultaneous increase in the consumption of sugar.

With the reduced mechanical stresses of chewing with industrial diets, there was less stimulation of the jaw muscles.

In other words, this is a relatively recent phenomenon linked to environmental factors. The increased prevalence of crooked teeth can be specifically traced to times and geographical areas where changes in diets have been introduced. It can even occur within just one generation. If it were a genetic phenomenon having something to do with natural selection and evolution, it would have taken a much longer time to become so common.

INFANT FEEDING PRACTICES

In addition, changes in infant feeding practices that came along with industrialisation have been proposed as another source for these troubles.

Fossil records indicate children in pre-industrialised populations were breastfed exclusively for six months, and then continued to be breastfed for a few years with the introduction of solids.[7]

With industrialisation, mothers worked out of the home in textile mills for the first time, and there was the introduction of commercial infant formulas and artificial nipples and pacifiers. After four to six months of exclusive bottle feeding, babies were weaned with soft, pureed and processed commercial baby foods well into the second year of life.

Some of these very soft foods do not need to be chewed and are instead sucked. This changes the swallow pattern, increasing the activity of the facial muscles. The muscles pull backward and inwards, further compounding the issue of poor forward facial development

In Part II, you will find out more about why breastfeeding is the most powerful workout for the muscles and is the number one factor we can modify to influence jaw development in the peak window of growth. You will learn about the importance of introducing texture earlier when introducing solids and why we must minimise pacifier use.

We know that diet consistency, chewing and breastfeeding can greatly impact the trajectory of jaw development, but what about what the muscles are doing during breathing?

ORAL REST POSTURE

Persistent, light forces can make a big impact, and what our muscles are doing at rest or during sleep, where we spend most of our time, has a bigger impact on the way we grow.

At rest, it is normal for the tongue to be lightly suctioned to the roof of the mouth where it can stimulate the midpalate suture and the development of the width of the palate. The lower jaw is postured closed and forwards, the lips are closed, and breathing is through the nose.

When the jaw's muscles are not developed properly through chewing hard, fibrous foods, they become slack, and the jaw and lips tend to drop open. The tongue is no longer able to stimulate proper development of the width of the palate and the face grows in a more downward and backward direction.

This has been compounded by a shift from hunting and gathering to a more sedentary lifestyle and a focus on living and working indoors. With industrialisation, we are more prone to allergies from pets, dust, and mold. Children are also now exposed early in life to daycare centres, which have been described as 'viral sinks.'[8] These allergies and chronic nasal congestion have exacerbated the problem of open mouths and weak musculature.

The following is a well-known case study presented by orthodontist Dr John Mew that highlights a problem that's occurring in epidemic proportions. It's about a boy who had good facial development which deteriorated after he was given a pet gerbil for his birthday, a change that led to chronic nasal congestion. He adapted by shifting to an open mouth posture which, in turn, led to a vertical growth pattern where his jaws no longer projected forward. Dr John Mew's son and fellow orthodontist Dr Mike Mew describes this phenomenon as "melting of the human face."

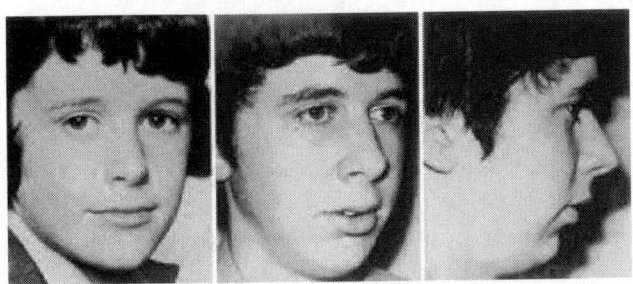

Shared and used with permission by Dr John Mew

In the well-researched book *Jaws: The story of a hidden epidemic*, evolutionist Paul Ehrlich and orthodontist Dr Sandra Kahn do a wonderful job of highlighting the epidemic of breathing problems and major health challenges related to shrinking jaws and crooked teeth.[9]

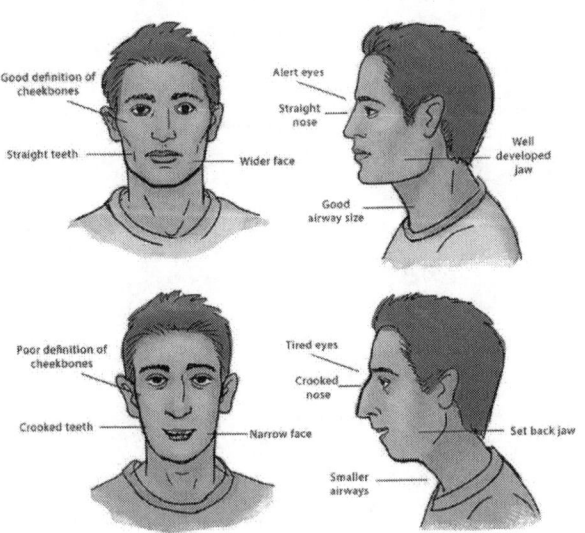

Shared and used with permission by Dr Sandra Kahn (*Jaws: The story of a hidden epidemic*, Stanford University Press)

THE PATH FORWARD IS OPTIMIZING ORAL FUNCTIONS

Understanding the evolution of shrinking jaws and the reduced functional demands associated with modern living allows us greater insights into a better path forward to alter the course of jaw development, breathing, and health.

All these issues point to a change in the way we are using our muscles, and form follows function. We need the correct functional stimulus for the face and jaws to grow properly. One of the most important muscles is the tongue. It is a very important muscle for the space it occupies.

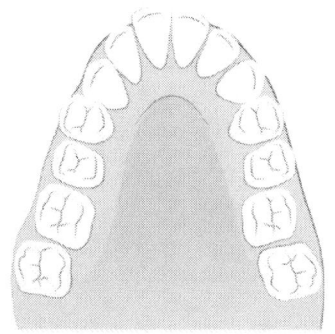
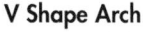
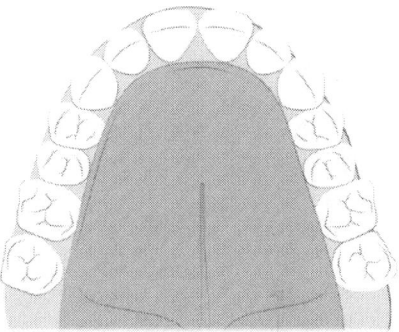

| V Shape Arch | U Shape Arch |

As I mentioned earlier, oral rest posture during the day and during sleep is influential because it is the light forces applied throughout the most substantial periods of time that have the biggest impact. The tongue should be lightly suctioned to the roof of the mouth at rest.

In this position, it forms the scaffold for normal palate development and counteracts the inward pressures of the lips and cheeks.

When this occurs, the palate will develop to perfectly house the tongue. This is similar to the skull growing around the brain or the orbit around the eye. It should be a perfect fit.

If the tongue drops for any reason including allergies, open mouth breathing, use of pacifiers, tongue-tie, low tone e.g. – prematurity, neuromuscular conditions – then there is nothing to counteract the inward pressures of the lips and cheeks, and the palate develops narrowly.

From a different perspective– when the tongue sits low, the force from the lips and cheeks prevails and causes distortion – leading to a high arch palate and a narrow nasal floor.

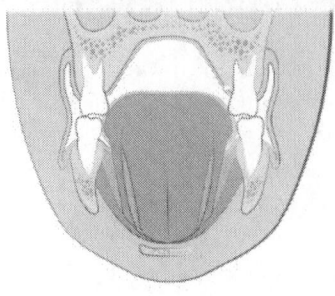 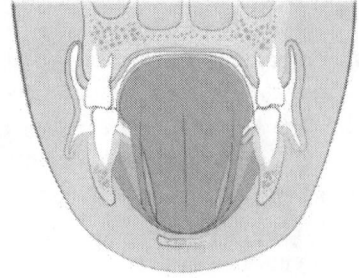

Poor Posture   **Good Posture**

Compare this to the tongue and palate being in intimate contact on the right. The palate and nasal passages are broad, and the tongue is well toned, and able to perform its most important function optimally – keeping the upper airway open during sleep.

The four elements of good oral rest posture:

- Tongue lightly suctioned to roof of mouth
- Lips gently sealed without strain
- Nasal breathing
- No activity of the muscles around the mouth during subconscious swallowing

PROPER FUNCTIONAL STIMULATION

In addition to achieving closed mouth nasal breathing and tongue suction at rest, it is important to stimulate proper muscle function during sucking, swallowing, and speech, especially in the under-six age group when the facial structures are growing most rapidly.[10,11]

> **It is important to stimulate proper muscle function during sucking, swallowing, and speech, especially in the under-six age group when the facial structures are growing most rapidly.**

This includes promoting good breastfeeding and latching during infancy and introducing foods that require chewing from around the age of six months versus overdoing purees. We also want to avoid habits like pacifier sucking, finger or thumb sucking, or prolonged sippy cup use.

Poor functional stimulation of bony development can begin in utero – for example, with prematurity or tongue-ties.[10,11]

Fetal echography studies have found that the third trimester is when the fetus has the most significant sucking and swallowing training in-utero. When a baby is born prematurely, they miss a significant period of muscle training. They often have lower tone, and this is compounded using nasogastric feeding tubes for them to feed, meaning they end up missing out on the mechanical benefits of early breastfeeding.

Long term follow-up studies of premature babies (excluding those who were fed by nasogastric tube) from Taiwan link prematurity to high arch palates and the development of mouth breathing and Obstructive Sleep Apnoea.[12] Reduced developmental outcomes and OSA have been linked to the high arch palate. In addition, when oral exercises were introduced to one cohort to help their tongue and mouth work more normally, they were more likely to have normalization of palate structures.

Modern medicine is a miracle. Not only can these premature babies survive and flourish, but we can help them thrive further by recognizing them as a high-risk group and addressing the specific risk factors of reduced oral tone, narrow palate, and mouth breathing early.

The other area which has had a lot of attention is tongue-ties. When the fold of tissue joining the undersurface of the tongue to the floor of the mouth is abnormally short or tight, it restricts normal mobility. This alters sucking and swallowing in-utero, and recent evidence supports an association between reduced tongue mobility and under-development of the palate.

Modern living makes it harder for us to express our full genetic potential in terms of jaw development, but my aim here is to help you understand the various risk factors so that we can strike as many different pins as possible.

MYOFUNCTIONAL DISORDERS AS EARLY WARNING SIGNS

Any time the muscles of the mouth and face don't work correctly – including during suction, swallowing, breathing, speech, and chewing – it is called a myofunctional disorder.

Form follows function. This means that even before crooked teeth and orthodontic problems become apparent, these dysfunctions are the earliest warning signs there will be issues.

Myofunctional disorders include:

- open mouth breathing
- problems with infant latching or sucking
- poor swallowing and excessive intake of air and reflux-like symptoms in infancy
- tongue-ties
- use of pacifiers, finger sucking
- overuse of bottles, sippy cups, and pouch foods
- nasal obstruction, enlarged adenoids and tonsils
- allergies and nasal congestion
- poor swallowing and eustachian tube clearance – recurrent ear infections, glue ear
- soft, overly processed diets
- difficulties with chewing and swallowing food
- messy, open mouth chewing
- drooling
- snoring
- teeth grinding or clenching
- speech delay
- lisps or speech misarticulations
- nail biting
- chewing on clothes, hair, and objects

We need all early child health professionals to start recognizing these as the earliest markers of airway problems and help set up children to develop optimal airway function and structure.

> **The most important thing you can do is be an advocate for your child's airway health.**

The following chapters will aid you with the knowledge and education to speak and act confidently on what your child may need to have evaluated.

PART II

EARLY CHILDHOOD INFLUENCES ON AIRWAY DEVELOPMENT

3

MOUTH BREATHING

Breathing – it's the most important thing that we do. We can last for days without water and food, but without air we can't last for more than a few minutes. Despite this fact, the importance of healthy nasal breathing isn't widely emphasized.

We are currently experiencing a hidden epidemic of mouth breathing. Research has shown that over 50% of preschool children breathe through their mouth.[1] But the bigger problem is that seeing children with their lips slightly separated or even hanging wide open is not something that many parents and health care professionals give a second thought about.

Nasal breathing has many distinct advantages over mouth breathing for dental, general, and sleep health across all ages, but it's particularly important for parents to pay attention to because the way a child breathes is an important influence on how their jaw and facial structures develop.

Form follows function, and in upcoming chapters we will discuss how breastfeeding, addressing tongue-ties, discouraging pacifiers, and encouraging good chewing can all help keep jaw and facial growth and development on track. But it is the *gentle forces* of the muscles during rest, and particularly during sleep, that have the most important effects, as they are acting for the greatest length of time. Nasal breathing, with the lips sealed and tongue up, promotes optimal muscle tone and balance and is therefore crucial.

> **When mouth breathing is not addressed early, the impact on poor facial and airway development will tip a child onto a downhill slide that leads to side effects like poorer breathing, sleep, and health into adulthood.**

In addition, chronic mouth breathing is a myofunctional disorder. It alters the way the tongue and other muscles of the mouth and face work, and is a catapult into picky eating, chewing and swallowing issues, and speech concerns.

Parents are not taught to connect the dots and identify mouth breathing as a root cause of other issues. What often happens instead is I'll see children with a whole bunch of symptoms that are being treated individually – behavioural or learning concerns, prolonged bedwetting, little progress with extended speech therapy, decay despite good diet and home care, and crooked teeth. Mouth breathing as a common contributor to all remains unaddressed.

In this chapter, I'm going to further outline the wide-ranging risks and consequences of continual mouth breathing – all of which are good reasons to pay attention to how your child is breathing.

Babies are born obligate nasal breathers, but I am seeing far too many infants in my practice with their lips gently apart at rest and their tongues sitting low. This tells me they are on track to become mouth breathers even before their first birthday.

George Caitlin, author of a book called *Shut Your Mouth and Save Your Life,* observed how the Native Americans had fantastic health and were in physically good condition compared to those in other societies.[2] They had fine teeth and beautiful faces, and he was convinced that these developed from careful attention to ensuring breathing with the mouth closed from the earliest days of life. For example, he noted Native American women gently withdrawing their nipples from the mouths of their infants and carefully closing the lips with their fingers. This is a simple thing we can look for and do from the moment a child is born.

More recently, journalist James Nestor released a widely acclaimed book called *Breath: The new science of a lost art.*[3] It's a well-researched book on how proper nasal breathing is becoming a missing pillar of health. He describes how, "no matter what you eat, how much you exercise, how skinny or young or wise you are, none of it matters if you're not breathing properly."

James shares how mouth breathing can be linked to snoring, allergies, asthma, auto-immune diseases, and anxiety. Through learning about the decline in jaw structures from ancient and pre-industrial times to modern times, he finds answers to the question of when breathing went wrong and explores how we can reclaim our health by adjusting the way we breathe.

James also subjected himself to mouth breathing for 10 days to see how quickly the change could impact health. Under the supervision of Professor Jayakar Nayak from Stanford Otolaryngology, he placed foam ear plugs in his nose, which forced him to breathe continuously through his mouth as he took measurements to assess the impact. He used a pulse-oximeter to measure heart rate and blood oxygen levels, and a phone app to get an indication of breathing at night.

He reported an increase in snoring from a couple of minutes per night to four hours per night within three days. He developed obstructive sleep apnoea. His blood pressure increased by an average of 13 points, putting him in the category of Stage 1 hypertension. His heart rate variability, which is a measure of nervous system balance, plummeted, reflecting a state of stress along with his increased pulse and reduced body temperature. James describes how his mental clarity hit rock bottom, and through this experiment he was beginning to feel like he hated life and each new day felt like Groundhog Day.

These drastic results – achieved in such a brief period – ensure that we can only imagine how children will suffer (both in the short- and long-term scheme of things) when they are breathing through their mouths for months or years at a time. Luckily, this is something we can have some control over. By restoring nasal breathing, we are also restoring a child's future potential.

Many times, when I first identify a child as a mouth breather, their parents are surprised to learn that there is a problem with this. After all, it's normalized in magazine shoots of models with their lips apart, and we're even told at the gym we're not working hard enough if we are not breathing through our mouth to get air.

The nose is specially designed for breathing; breathing through our mouth should become as abnormal as eating or speaking with our nose.

A BRIEF REVIEW OF NASAL ANATOMY

Inside the nasal cavity, there are three-per-side sausage-shaped projections of bone-covered mucous membranes called the superior, middle, and inferior turbinates. These convoluted projections of bone slow airflow and allow it to be properly warmed to body temperature, humidified, and filtered before it enters our lungs. The mucous membrane lining the nose traps and collects bacteria and filters particles such as dust and pollen. It also slightly moistens the air as it passes, reducing dehydration.

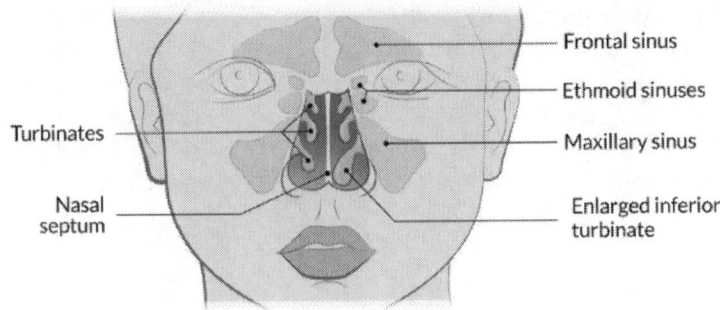

A further, often overlooked, advantage of nasal breathing relates to nitric oxide. This is formed and released in the para-nasal sinuses, and when air is inhaled through the nose, it gets more nitric oxide. Nitric oxide has antimicrobial properties and sterilises the air as it enters the lower respiratory tract. It is also a potent vasodilator, which means that as air is inhaled into the lungs, the blood vessels in the alveoli expand. This allows a greater volume of blood to pass through as well as more efficient uptake and circulation of oxygen throughout the body.

THE CONSEQUENCES OF MOUTH BREATHING

Most of us can understand what it is like to have a stuffy nose when we have a cold. It affects our sleep, energy, and function. But mainstream healthcare neglects nasal breathing as a key pillar of health and disease progression, and many health professionals remain unaware of the wide-ranging consequences. In children, some of these are irreversible. Here's what to look out for:

Dry mouth. This can lead to chapped lips, bad breath, increased risk of dental disease including decay, and inflamed gums due to reduced protective effects of saliva.

Increased risks of upper airway problems. With mouth breathing, air bypasses this first line of defense, and children are more prone to upper airway infections and irritation and enlargement of the adenoids and tonsils. Problems include rhinitis, sinusitis, ear infections, and increased use of antibiotics in childhood.[4] Mouth breathing has also been found to be an independent risk factor for asthma and this is likely an extension of upper airway inflammation into the lungs.[5]

Altered tongue posture and the development of other myofunctional disorders. Chronic mouth breathing is a myofunctional disorder, which means it alters the way the muscles of the mouth, face, and airway rest and function.[6,7] It is associated with tongue thrust or lowered tongue posture and low orofacial muscle tone. These have a knock-on effect on other functions including altered chewing, swallowing, and speech.

Accompanying alterations during the functions of chewing, swallowing, and speech functions include:

- picky eating or a preference for soft foods
- open mouth chewing
- the tongue thrusting between the teeth during swallowing to help form
- seal if the lips can't close
- inability to swallow food or pouching of foods
- the need for liquids to help swallow during meals
- choking during mealtimes
- excess tension of the muscles of the lips
- lisps or poor clarity of speech sounds, particularly with n, l, t, d, s, and z sounds

Poor facial development. Due to the chronic changes in muscle posture and tone, there is reduced functional stimulus for the jaws to grow properly.[8] Adenoid facies or "long face syndrome" may develop. This is just one of the most common patterns of altered facial development that occurs with chronic mouth breathing. It is characterized by sunken eyes, narrow, pinched nostrils, open mouth, a narrow high arch palate, crooked teeth, protruding upper teeth, and an everted upper lip. With a slack lower jaw, the face tends to grow long and backwards, and the airway becomes pinched. The narrow high palate and receded jaws become risk factors for disturbed breathing and sleep into adulthood.

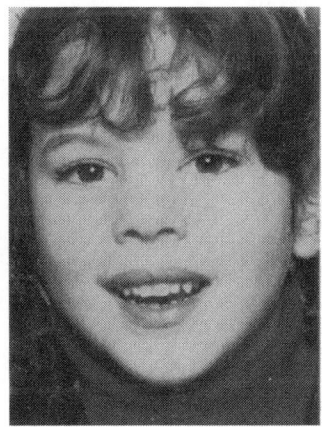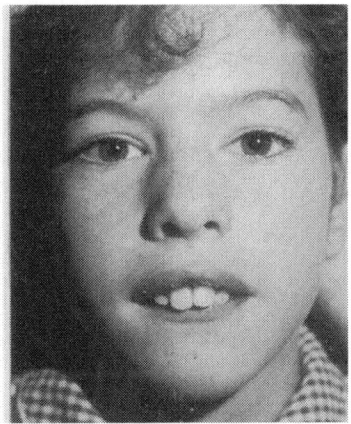

Supplied and used with permission by Dr John Mew

When nasal obstruction is relieved relatively early in life, there is greater likelihood of a return to a closed mouth default and a normalised facial appearance. At the same time, if it is not addressed, it may leave an indelible mark on the structure of the face.[9]

Crooked teeth. This reflects the underlying deficiency in jaw development. If mouth breathing is not properly attended to, it continues to be a common cause of relapse or instability of results post-orthodontic treatment.

Sleep disturbed breathing. Mouth breathing increases resistance to airflow in the upper airway by 2.5 times.[10] This increases airway collapsibility and risk of snoring and OSA leading to unrestorative sleep. Do this little exercise at home: try snoring with your mouth open and then again with your mouth closed. You should notice when your mouth is closed air flows more smoothly and there is less vibration of the soft palate and therefore a lessened sound of snoring. When air flows more freely, it takes less effort to breathe, and the throat and upper airway are less likely to collapse. When the mouth is open and the jaw is slack, the tongue is more likely to sit low and fall back into the throat. These breathing difficulties rob children of the full restorative benefits of sleep.

Increased risk of behavioural, socio-emotional, and learning problems. The experience of unrestorative sleep in children may manifest as poor attention or hyperactivity, and symptoms may mimic ADHD.[11] A recent study of 100 primary school-aged mouth breathing children found the most common symptom of inattention was "failing to give close attention during school." This affected 73% of children.[12] It's important to investigate mouth breathing before children are medicated. In two separate studies of 11,000 children by Bonuck and team, mouth breathing in the earliest years of life was established as an independent risk factor for the development of behavioural and socio-emotional problems at age four and seven years[13], and the likelihood that a child will have special education needs at age eight years.[14]

Sensory processing disorders. Our brain relies on sensory information to organize, prioritise, understand, and respond to our environment. Sensory processing disorders refer to when the sensory information from hearing, vision, taste, smell, touch, pressure, and movements is misinterpreted and does not get organized into appropriate responses. This can lead to difficulties with motor activities, transitions, and sequenced tasks, and can hinder children's ability to succeed with everyday activities and normal social participation.

A high concentration of sensory receptors is found in our lips, tongue, and nose. Therefore, it is not surprising that when function is altered by mouth breathing, there may be issues with sensory processing.

New research is finding that children who breathe through their mouths may have double the risk of sensory processing disorders.[15]

Something related, which I have developed a strong interest in recently, is the link between tics and breathing. Tics are sudden twitches, movements or sounds people do repeatedly, without any control. Whilst only small numbers so far, I've found it remarkable to see reduction in facial tics with children who have practiced deep nasal breathing or with improved airflow during palate expansion and have since discovered compelling research that supports this.[16]

There's still a lot to be discovered in this area, but it's another very important reason to pay attention to nasal breathing from infancy.

Changes in body posture.[17] These may be adopted to help with the smooth passage of air. Forward head posture may occur – where the head and lower jaw are projected forward, leading to changes in the neck and shoulders. Rather than the weight of the head (equivalent to the weight of a bowling ball) being distributed down the whole body, it is supported solely by the neck and shoulders, which can lead to chronic neck tension. Some researchers have even documented that to keep the body in balance there may be alterations in the curvature of the spine and distant changes in the feet.

WHAT CAUSES MOUTH BREATHING?

The most commonly recognisable factors contributing to mouth breathing are allergic rhinitis, enlarged adenoids and tonsils, and deviated septums.

Allergic rhinitis is the most common factor to be associated with mouth breathing. This is an allergic reaction causing the swelling of the nasal lining as a reaction to airborne allergens such as pollen, dust mites, animal fur, and mold. One of the larger studies of mouth breathing in children aged three to nine years found that 81.4% had allergic rhinitis, testing positive to at least one allergen on skin testing.[18] In contrast, when the children had the internal passage of their airway assessed with a nasal endoscope, enlarged adenoids were only present in 37.6% and enlarged tonsils in 12.6%. While 72.1% of children had a deviated septum, only 1% had deviations that could be considered obstructive. This study reinforces that we need to be paying more attention to allergies, including when other nasal surgeries are offered.

Allergic rhinitis and other childhood allergies have their origins in gestation. Common influences include exposure to cigarette smoke, maternal obesity, stress, depression, environmental pollution, reduced vitamin D and sun exposure, skin dryness and more.

The atopic march refers to a natural progression of allergic diseases that often occurs in childhood. It begins with eczema or food allergies (including dairy, egg, and nuts) in infancy, to asthma and allergic rhinitis later in childhood. Each of these allergies is often managed individually with different specialists.

I am beginning to pay more attention to those early signs of allergies, as they may be a sign that a child will have an increased risk of developing allergic rhinitis and nasal congestion down the track.

To help offset these early signs, parents can take simple actions to reduce the probability of allergic rhinitis symptoms in their children. For example, minimizing dust exposure through washing bed sheets regularly, reducing the number of soft toys in bed, keeping pets out of the bedroom, or starting a regular practice of nasal clearing with saline or medicated sprays twice per day in the same period that they brush their teeth. The more we can do to keep allergies at bay before the symptoms of chronic nasal congestion and obstruction appear, the better.

Enlarged adenoids and tonsils are a common contributor to obstructive breathing – these will be discussed further in Chapter 8, where I will also present an alternative view that sometimes those problems could have their origin in nasal disuse. You see, the more we use the nose, the easier it becomes to breathe clearly through it.

Nasal disuse.

> We need to differentiate if a child has true nasal obstruction or merely the perception of obstruction that comes from congestion and nasal disuse despite an adequate nasal airway, as surgeries will not be effective in reducing that perception.

Open mouth breathing could also be a habit or pattern learned from watching family members, so it's important to take note if you breathe with your mouth as well.

One thing to do before jumping into surgery in conjunction with a trained medical professional is to see how comfortably your child can breathe with their lip sealed for a few minutes. ENT surgeon Dr Soroush Zaghi and team published a study to support the idea that, if a child could be observed breathing comfortably with their lips sealed for three minutes using Micropore (porous) tape, or with water in their mouth, it was worthwhile doing nasal clearing exercises and nasal breathing practices to improve symptoms before proceeding with surgery.[19]

Narrow palates. The whole problem of nasal obstruction can be compounded by or even have its origins in narrow palates. The palate is the floor of the nose. Narrow palates are linked to narrow nasal passages and increased resistance to normal nasal airflow. Mouth breathing may be adopted in compensation, therefore setting off a downhill spiral of poor tongue posture and poor palate development. There are times when a child's jaw structures become too small for the tongue to fit properly; at this point it becomes difficult for children to close their mouth. We will go into more detail later palate expansion and widening as an effective option to promote nasal breathing, and the need for greater integration between ENTs and dental professionals to restore nasal breathing.

> **Narrow palates are linked to narrow nasal passages and increased resistance to normal nasal airflow.**

RESTORING NASAL BREATHING FOR CHILDREN

By the time a child has nasal surgery or palate expansion to address poor nasal airflow, they are most likely to have already been mouth breathers for at least six months and interventions will not automatically lead to nasal breathing. There is altered resting tone of the oral and facial muscles which will need to be addressed to return to nasal breathing during sleep, including restoring proper lip seal, normal tongue tone, and tongue to palate sealing. Addressing any tongue-ties and utilizing myofunctional therapy will be important pieces of the puzzle to solve this issue. We'll talk more about these topics in Chapters 5 and 10.

I'm particularly interested in learning more about the role of breathing re-education and re-training a child to breathe deeply through their belly or diaphragm as opposed to shallow and through their upper chest muscles. We are starting to understand that this is important for optimal breathing during sleep in many different ways. Diaphragmatic breathing stimulates the vagus nerve, which sends a signal to the body to relax and de-stress. You can also practice this with your child with a breathing app like One Deep Breath, or you can read more on Buteyko breathing and how it can help manage conditions like allergies, asthma, sleep apnoea, and anxiety from breathing re-educator and author Patrick McKeown.

The earlier mouth breathing is addressed, the simpler the treatment. We will go through this in more detail in part two, but for now, here is a rough summary: it will take a team approach to address all risk factors.

Help spread the word that nasal breathing is an important key pillar of health and needs to be the goal – even after procedures like ENT surgery or orthodontic treatment.[20,21] Without nasal breathing, children will not be able to live up to their full potential.

> **When mouth breathing goes unaddressed in the critical early years of facial development, it leaves a permanent mark on their facial development and alters a child's trajectory of breathing, sleep, learning, and total health.**

We need to identify mouth breathing early and work in teams with ENTs, allergy, dental, and speech specialists; myofunctional therapists, physical therapists, breathing re-educators and more to address all the obstructive, structural, muscle, and behavioural components and their consequences. Let's call this movement "Inspiration by Integration," a phrase coined by good friend and colleague Stanford Sleep Surgeon Dr Stanley Liu, who co-hosted a multi-disciplinary sleep conference with this title in Melbourne with me in February 2020. Despite all the innovation he has been responsible for in advanced jaw reconstructive surgery to help adults with obstructive sleep apnoea breathe better, he has also been a passionate advocate for early intervention, including the promotion of nasal breathing in childhood.

In the next chapter, I'll introduce how the way we feed our infants can have important implications on how they breathe decades down the track.

INFANT FEEDING AND SUCKING HABITS

The way we feed our babies and how we introduce food in the first year of life are other important influences on how their muscles work and jaws grow. The first year of life is especially significant because this is the window of most rapid development of jaw and facial structures.

Many of us already know breastfeeding is linked with several long-term health benefits for both babies and mothers. Numerous studies have focused on the nutritional and immunological benefits of breastmilk. It is perfectly made by nature, and its composition throughout feeds and as babies grow can change in order to provide precisely what babies need.

However, less promoted are the *mechanical* benefits of feeding at the breast and the development of normal orofacial muscle patterns compared to bottle feeding. This is why even expressed breastmilk fed through a bottle isn't quite the same.

My involvement with airway problems began with offering adults with snoring and obstructive sleep apnoea dental devices that held their jaw forward during sleep to open their airways. It made me question why we couldn't just get the jaws to grow properly in the first place.

I was at a conference in 2014 when paediatric dentist and author of "Early Treatment of Malocclusions: Prevention and Interception in Primary Dentition", Dr German Ramirez, shared that breastfeeding is the single most important influence that can help stimulate proper lower jaw development in the first year of life. This was my initial inspiration to become a passionate advocate of the mechanical benefits of breastfeeding, and why I ultimately decided to become involved in tongue-tie release for infants with breastfeeding challenges.

Breastfeeding requires a complex co-ordination of the tongue, jaw, and other orofacial muscles to suck, swallow, and breathe. This makes it a process with an essential role in preparing the muscles for future functions (like speaking and chewing) in addition to its importance relating to proper facial development.

Ultrasound research by Donna Geddes and the team at the University of Australia demonstrated that optimal transfer of milk occurs via tongue suction.[1]

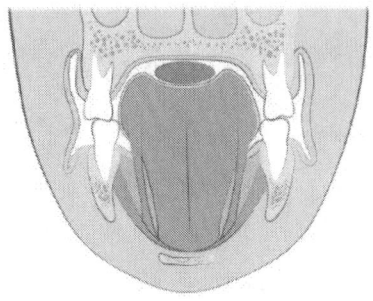 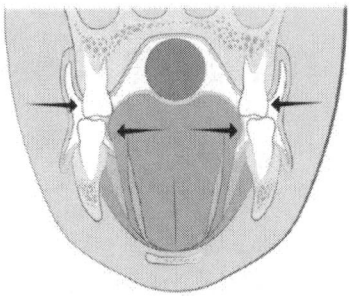

Tongue position while breastfeeding **Tongue position while bottle feeding**

The tongue must suction firmly against the roof of the mouth. As it lowers, it creates a vacuum that expands the ducts in the breast and promotes the flow of milk from the breast into the infant's mouth.

> **As the tongue elevates and presses the breast tissue against the palate, it also helps to sculpt the palate and nasal passages, making them wide and broad. This explains why breastfeeding is sometimes referred to as "nature's palate expander."**

Meanwhile, with bottle feeding, the artificial teat is not as malleable and therefore does not allow for proper molding of the palate. It alters the tongue posture, and rather than the infant being able to control the flow of milk, it tends to come out more easily with use of the lips and cheeks. The excessive inward forces of the lips and cheeks narrow the jaws and reduce space for proper tongue-to-palate seal at rest and the future teeth. The net result is a distortion of the hard palate and the nasal airway directly above it.

Breastfeeding also helps the jaws and face grow forward. The lower jaw forms the stable basis for tongue movements, and its movements help to create the intraoral pressure changes during feeding. As the lower jaw moves backwards and forwards, it stimulates the lower jaw joint cartilage. This is a growth centre, which means new bone is deposited there, resulting in forward growth.

At the start of each suck, the lower jaw and tongue rise, and the tip of the tongue pushes the areola and nipple against the front part of the hard palate, behind where the front teeth will sit in the future. This stimulates the incisive suture or pre-maxillary suture, providing the stimulus for the forward development of the upper jaw and cheekbones. Paediatric dentist and dental anthropologist Dr Kevin Boyd describes the action of the tongue as being like a piston that pushes the whole midface forward.

This powerful co-ordination of muscles drives the proper development of the face. As the jaws and face grow forward, so does the airway.

Research suggests that six months of breastfeeding is associated with a reduction of the probability of orthodontic problems developing, such as overbites, open bites, and posterior crossbites with the baby teeth.[2-4] This effect may be even greater if breastfeeding is continued beyond six months. It's important to connect that these orthodontic problems are most often a reflection or symptom of poor jaw and airway development.

The other thing to be aware of is that pacifier use can negate the protective effects of breastfeeding.

Peres and team compared the impact of exclusive and predominant breastfeeding and the impact of pacifier use and assessed the presence of orthodontic problems at age five.[5]

The group found that 'exclusive breastfeeding' was protective against orthodontic problems by the age of five years, regardless of whether a pacifier was used. In contrast when were 'predominantly breastfed' there was less of a protective effect when pacifiers were used.

Breastfeeding also allows a baby to control the rate of milk transfer and co-ordinate their sucking, swallowing, and breathing. They can feed and maintain nasal breathing simultaneously. In contrast, as mentioned previously, milk flows out of a bottle easily. Different teat sizes and flows are prescribed for different ages. As milk comes out rapidly from the bottle, the baby must take pauses to breathe. This is where mouth breathing begins. It's harder to co-ordinate sucking, swallowing, and breathing in the same way as with breastfeeding.

In summary, good breastfeeding with proper positioning:

- requires a complex co-ordination of all the muscles of the mouth and face to suck, swallow and breathe
- is a powerful muscle workout compared to bottle feeding
- prepares the muscles for good chewing, swallowing and speech sounds[6,7]
- utilizes tongue suction which helps develop the tongue tone required for tongue-to-palate seal at rest and optimal nasal breathing
- provides the proper functional stimulus for optimal development of our jaw bones, or bony support of the airway[8,9]

Bottle feeding is an alteration of normal muscle patterns and is more likely to lead to other dysfunctions as a child grows. If we understand the importance of optimal function, then there are actions that we can take proactively for bottle-fed children to help get function and structure back on track early.

For all these benefits to be expressed, we need to look beyond ensuring feeding is pain free and resulting in good weight gain. We must pay special attention to achieving an effective, deep latch.

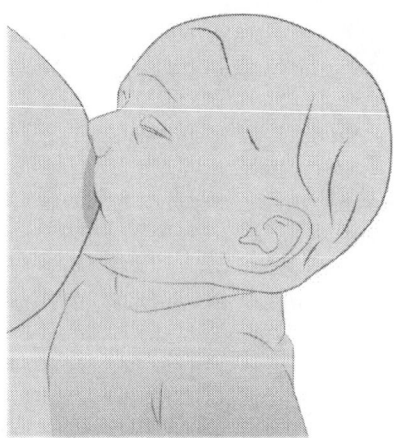 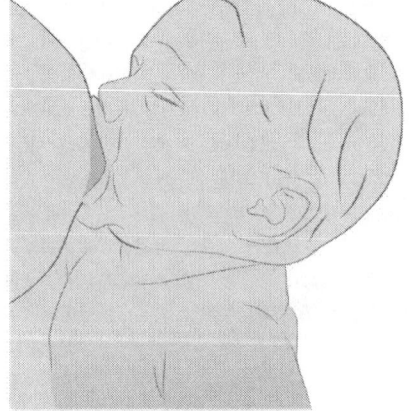

Shallow latch   Deep latch

A good latch should not only be comfortable, but it should be deep. This allows proper function of the tongue and other muscles. It is still possible to have a shallow and pain-free latch with good weight gain, but the infant will be overusing their lips and cheeks to extract milk. An International Board-Certified Lactation Consultant (IBCLC) is usually the most qualified person to help check the positioning and latch and give you feedback.

A poor, shallow latch may be painful, as a baby uses their lips, cheeks, and gums to extract milk and will be less effective at doing so. This may be incorrectly perceived as low milk supply or frustration at the breast – especially around the age of three months when milk supply becomes less hormonally driven and is stimulated by the demand or rate of transfer from the breast.

We also need to be alert to the possibility of a tongue-tie, which is something every baby should be checked for at birth. This should involve the paediatrician physically lifting the tongue up and getting an indication if the attachment between the tongue and floor of the mouth is unusually short or tight. As alterations may be subtle, tongue-ties cannot always be definitively diagnosed on the spot, but parents should be made aware that the issue could express itself more fully and contribute to other problems later in development. The next chapter will cover tongue-ties in more detail.

After working with many babies, I am a big advocate for craniosacral therapy or cranial osteopathy for babies after birth. Many babies have strains or misalignment in their head, neck, and other structures. This can be related to restriction of space in utero or can be related to the birth process. Babies with fast or traumatic deliveries or interventions including c-sections, vacuums, and forceps may be at risk. These therapies unwind areas of general body tension and restriction, relieve compression in the head region, and reduce impingement or optimize function of important cranial nerves that reside in the skull. These nerves are involved in the co-ordination of sucking, swallowing, breathing, and movement of the tongue.

Inevitably, when I bring up the mechanical benefits of breastfeeding among health care professionals, I end up hearing differing opinions on the divisive topic – with some professionals suggesting 'breast is best' and others suggesting 'fed is best'. We certainly don't want to make mums feel guilty and create additional anxiety that overwhelms them.

However, the parents that are most prone to guilt are those that really want to breastfeed and are struggling without effective knowledge or answers to address their challenges from their health care professionals. The distribution of formula samples to doctors and their easy availability to families is not the solution.

There is a great need to highlight the mechanical benefits of breastfeeding to parents and professionals. This will ensure that parents can make the most fully informed decisions – even before birth – and professionals can give the best advice and support.

Quite often, well-intended professional advice can be a barrier to a good start to breastfeeding. For example, the first hour of life is considered the 'golden hour' where babies should ideally be left on the breast undisturbed. This helps with attachment, increased prolactin and oxytocin hormone levels, and the baby's first bolus of colostrum. Videos demonstrate a breast crawl, which is when a baby is born and placed immediately on their mother's chest, where they instinctively crawl from the tummy up to their mother's nipple looking for their first feed. Babies who can start feeding by themselves this way are less likely to have problems breastfeeding.

But there are a lot of checks that happen in the hospital, and the separation of babies from their mothers occurs with the medicalisation of births. Personally, my first daughter was delivered via emergency C-section and was born with a fever. She was taken away immediately without encouraging a feed. I was persuaded by hospital staff to rest up, and formula was introduced within the first day of her life without me knowing any better that my milk coming in would be impacted. I came away from the hospital thinking it was very acceptable to supplement with formula and bought the same bottles and formula offered in the hospital.

I ultimately ended up dropping formula and maintained breastfeeding until six months. But I see so many mothers given incorrect information that hinders this goal.

If we want to make mothers feel less guilty, it is not by avoiding the promotion of breastfeeding. We need to separate mothers and babies less, offer better education and advice, and promote more skillful and knowledgeable professionals who can help mothers maintain their supply and help them overcome challenges.

I recommend Dr Jack Newman's *Guide to Breastfeeding* for any expectant or new mothers who want more information on breastfeeding.[10]

PACIFIERS

The use of pacifiers can be a source of conflicting advice and confusion for parents, as there are pros and cons on each side.

I didn't think I would offer my children pacifiers as a dentist, but as a new mother, I found it was helpful to offer one to my eldest daughter to get some extra peace and quiet time for a quick shower. Pacifier use was also reinforced by our child health nurse at the time. Fast forward to three years later, and she was still reliant on it to settle herself to sleep. I fully appreciate the benefits of pacifiers to help calm and settle babies and parents in turn, and that this can be a hard habit to break.

However, what I wish I had known then is that it's not just about the teeth, and there are lasting implications far beyond when the pacifier habit is kicked. It's important that you and all our infant and child health professionals understand the full impact of pacifiers on palate development and breathing down the track.

The pacifier, like the artificial teat on a bottle, alters the tongue's position and swallowing pattern so the tongue doesn't elevate and properly mold the roof of the mouth. Along with the inward pressures of the lips and cheeks, the palate is distorted. Children with pacifier use are known to have an increased risk of orthodontic problems with their baby teeth.

One of the biggest conflicts around advice to avoid pacifier use is that there is some research to suggest that it may be protective against sudden infant death syndrome (SIDS).[11]

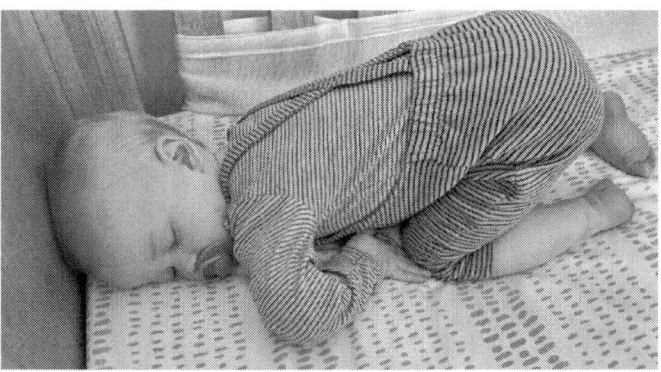

Parent photo used with consent

Stomach sleeping is the single most important risk factor that has been associated with sudden infant death syndrome, and it has been suggested that this group of children may be most protected.[12] Usually when I think of children lying on their stomachs, I wonder whether there is low tongue posture, which would mean their tongue is more likely to obstruct the airway during sleep when they are on their back. It has recently been proposed that sucking a pacifier creates a negative pressure that promotes the back of the tongue to form a seal with the soft palate and keep the airway open.[13]

I suspect that, in the future, we may find that these children who require a pacifier would be more directly served by improving the base of tongue mobility and tongue to palate suction, and by promoting breastfeeding, which has been found to be protective against SIDS.

Other demonstrated benefits of pacifier use include the reduction of perception of pain with surgical procedures and potentially aiding the organization of sucking reflexes in premature babies.

The cons of pacifiers can be summarized as follows:

- may create nipple confusion and interfere with the early establishment of breastfeeding
- increases the risk of orthodontic problems, most notably anterior open bites and posterior crossbites[14-16]

- can negate the protective effect of breastfeeding against orthodontic problems
- it is associated with increased risk of middle ear infections
- interferes with free tongue movement and the development of normal speech perception[17]
- interferes with facial mimicry or the imitation of perceived facial expressions – there is some evidence this can impact the development of empathy and emotional competence in some children in the long term[18]
- persistent changes in muscle function even after use is eliminated – these include increased likelihood of poor lip seal, low tongue posture or tongue thrust, open mouth breathing, and altered swallowing[19]

All the adverse consequences are related to the intensity, frequency, and duration of sucking. Minimizing use of the pacifier will reduce these risks. It also means that even if pacifiers are used only at night, there may still be considerable impacts due to the relatively long duration of time that children are asleep for.

There are no pacifier brands proven to protect against orthodontic issues.[20] In fact, a successful class action was filed against a company that is well known for their 'orthodontic' line of pacifiers.[21] These pacifiers were promoted as enhancing children's oral and orofacial development and presented as superior to conventional pacifiers and safe to use in children over 24 months in the absence of any supporting evidence. I would tend to go with a nipple that is flattest and will interfere least with proper tongue posture.

The general advice is that pacifier use is acceptable until the age of six months – but there is no scientific basis to this recommendation.

A baby's jaw is most moldable in the earliest years of life. Improper muscle balance will have the greatest detriment in this window.

While pacifier use can be a life-changer to help calm babies, it can also be a crutch. It is a good idea to identify the cause of the upset instead of always relying on a pacifier for calming the baby.

By age five to six months, babies develop more oral control and begin the process of discriminatory mouthing. It can be appropriate to introduce mouth toys for babies that help them explore more of the back of their mouth and not just the front. One of the simplest things I like to offer in favour of regular teethers is a baby toothbrush they can handle and insert deeper into their mouth. This helps babies develop sensory discrimination within the mouth that ultimately helps with food manipulation and speech.

The following photos below illustrate changes in the mouth and teeth that occurred in a five-month time frame where the patient discontinued pacifier use after a dental trauma. He also had therapy to improve his tongue's resting posture, co-ordination, and tone.

You can note the widening of the palate and rounding of the dental arch. His open bite has closed. There is, however, still a lack of normal spacing between his baby teeth, which indicates a deficit of jaw development and is a warning sign that the permanent teeth will be crowded.

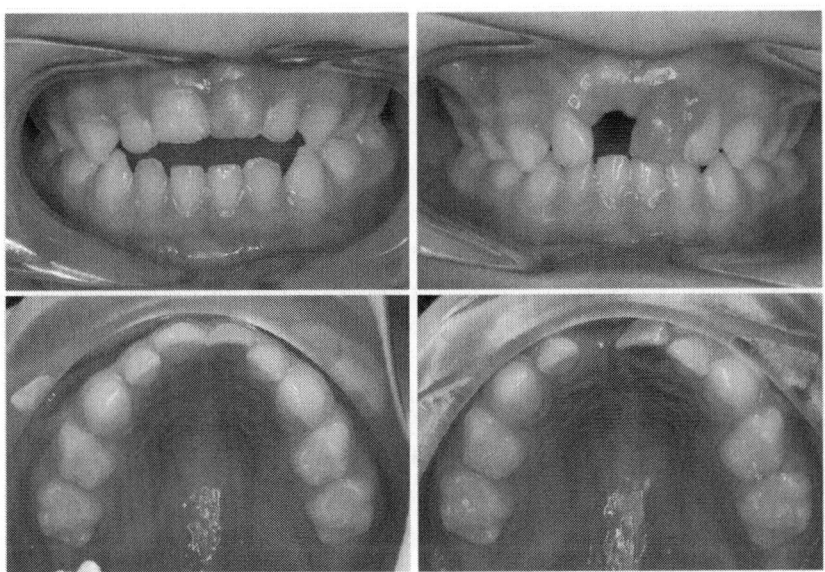

Still, this case effectively illustrates how the jaws structures are quite moldable in the early years of life. The dysfunctions of the muscles will readily distort the palate. At the same time, if the habit is discontinued early as possible, there is also greater potential for normalization of both the muscle habits and jaw and facial structures.

One of the common thoughts is that offering children a pacifier is better than digit sucking because a pacifier can be taken away from them. This is not supported by analysis of evidence pooled from multiple studies by Dogmaci and team from the University of Adelaide.[15] They found pacifier use was associated with an increased risk of crossbites (reflecting a narrow palate) whilst digit suckers were more likely to have increased overjet (reflecting some flaring of the upper front teeth and a receded lower jaw). Overall, they found that the pacifier use was associated with more significant issues.

For this reason, although it's commonly thought a pacifier is easier to replace than a thumb later down the track, I'm not convinced about the value of replacing a thumb sucking habit with a pacifier. Thumb sucking is a more active habit. Children tend to remove their thumbs when they are talking, reducing the duration of time a thumb is in the mouth.

Instead, I tend to see sucking habits as compensation for sub-optimal tongue function and airway problems. The over-reliance on these habits could be fulfilling an important need and may be an early warning sign to be proactive in restoring normal function as children grow.

Italian researcher Dr Ferrante has produced research that suggested that thumb or finger sucking plays an important role in neurotransmission.[22]

Thumb sucking stimulates an area at the front of the palate behind the teeth, also known as the "palatal spot." This area is full of sensory receptors for an important nerve called the trigeminal nerve. The thumb on the spot is like a switch that passes a signal through the nerve, to the brain. This results in the release of important neurotransmitters.[23] These include serotonin and dopamine, which are involved in a range of other functions including balance, mood control, concentration, attention, memory, helping to enter deep sleep, and prevention of depression.

Dr Ferrante was able to demonstrate that when children were encouraged to place their tongue on this spot at rest and during swallowing, their balance improved. Children with tongue-ties did not have the same improvements as children with no restriction of tongue mobility.

The implication is that thumb sucking is serving an important function, and that ceasing the habit without replacing it with good tongue posture may not lead to lasting results. It suggests that children who thumb suck should be assessed for restricted tongue-ties and airway problems that would lead to open mouth breathing and lowered tongue posture.

This research will help explain why in practice, when children are ready to give up the thumb sucking habit, there is most often very immediate and predictable success through a program of habit elimination and myofunctional therapy to retrain normal resting tongue posture.

This contrasts with many other common options that don't address the underlying need for stimulation. These include:

- positive reinforcement
- varnishes
- band-aids
- thumb sucking gloves
- thumb guards

When these solutions do not work, an anti-habit orthodontic appliance may be fixed in the mouth. These solutions use metal prongs or barriers that block the thumb from the mouth. Again, these do not address the root problem and may reduce space in the mouth for the tongue to rest and function correctly.

In some children, this may force their tongue backwards, encroaching upon the airway and impacting breathing and sleep.

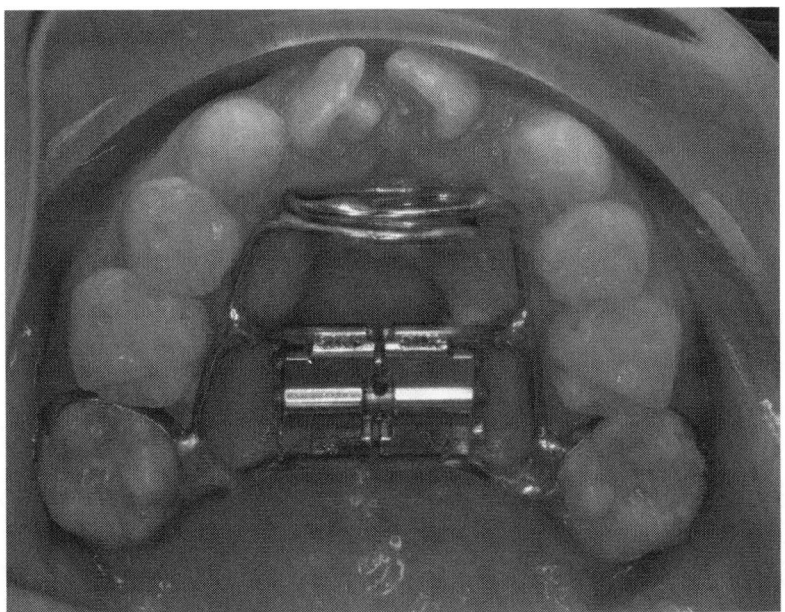

For children as young as six months, I would suggest looking into an oral appliance called a Bebe Munchee as a pacifier replacement during the day, even after the habit has ceased. This offers more appropriate functional stimulation of the oral and facial muscles.

Normal muscle patterns that I look to re-establish through myofunctional therapy for children with both sucking habits as they grow include:

- tongue resting lightly suctioned to the roof of the mouth
- lips closed at rest
- breathing through the nose day and night
- no movement of the facial muscles during swallowing

Even when these options are effective at habit elimination, tongue thrusts, and other myofunctional disorders, abnormal jaw development and orthodontic problems often persist.

Most orthodontic advice says not to worry much about thumb sucking until a child's permanent teeth come through around the age of seven years. The problem with this advice is that by this time the jaw structures will be less malleable, meaning some of the disturbances of development will have become more difficult to reverse.

Many parents recognise the development of these issues too late. They get concerned about their child's facial appearance, self-esteem, or risk of dental injuries only when the upper teeth protrude, the lower teeth are tipped back, and there is a big opening between the teeth that matches the thumb or finger.

It becomes hard for their child to seal their lips together easily and re-establish normal rest posture of the tongue, closed mouth nasal breathing, and proper swallowing.

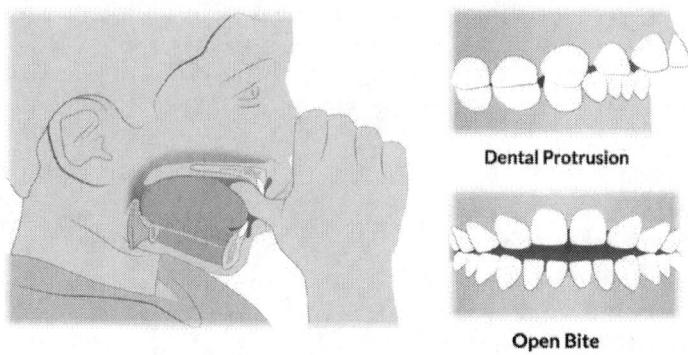

Dental Protrusion

Open Bite

> **The take-home message for children with a reliance on sucking habits, or any other associated and prolonged habits such as chewing on blankies or other objects such as shirt collars, nail biting, lip sucking, or drooling, is to see someone with expertise in myofunctional therapy early to identify the next window of opportunity to get things back on track.**

GOOD CHEWING PRACTICES

In the pre-industrial or indigenous populations, it was normal for children to be breastfed for up to three years with the gradual introduction of pre-chewed meat and tough fibrous foods. There were no naturally occurring purees.

Paediatric dentist and dental anthropologist Kevin Boyd and advocate for Baby Led Weaning says:

"It's called kiss feeding. Modern-day hunter-gatherers (there's not many of them left, but some aboriginal cultures still do these practices) will pre-chew the food like a bird does and spit it into the child's mouth. It sounds gross, but it's actually not. It's quite wonderful."

"Usually, by seven-, eight-, and certainly nine-months-old – even though a child didn't have that many, if any, teeth – they were chewing with their gums everything that anyone in the tribe was chewing. Certainly, by a year old, there was no difference in what a child ate from an adult. That would continue into the third year of life. Children were typically breastfed on demand while weaning onto firm, regular foods into the third year of life and sometimes beyond. That pattern is consistent throughout the human history."

Today, it is common for a baby's first solids to be pureed and introduced via a spoon. There is no evidence that spoon feeding purees is a helpful developmental stage for most babies. It is simply a shift that has occurred in modern societies.

Understanding how these cultural changes have contributed to reduced functional stimulus for strong jaw development offers a strategy to promote better function. Going back to introducing whole foods that require chewing (rather than introducing purees) resembles the natural feeding transition in paleolithic times, when dental crowding was rare.

Breastfeeding with an optimal latch offers the most powerful muscle workout of the chewing muscles, and research has shown us that this is associated with persistent gains in strength of all our chewing muscles.[7] By preschool age, those children who have breastfed will tend to have better chewing function with their mouth closed, appropriate jaw activity, and reduced activity of the facial muscles with chewing and swallowing.

> **While optimal muscle function begins with breastfeeding, Dr Gillian Rapley suggests that an approach to introducing solids called 'baby-led weaning' (BLW) continues this path.**

Dr Rapley completed PhD research comparing spoon- and self-feeding and is author of the book *Baby-Led Weaning: The essential guide to introducing solid foods*.[24] She noted that it was quite common for babies around the eight-month mark to experience problems like food refusal, picky eating, constipation (especially formula-fed babies), and choking on lumpier foods. She found that many of these challenges could be avoided by introducing self-feeding from the moment solids are introduced from six months, and during the transition from exclusively milk feeds to no milk.

Spoon feeding is associated with more rapid swallowing and decreased time of food in the mouth. It involves minimal jaw movements and there is a tendency to suck foods, which can lead to a persistent immature swallow. Functionally, the result is increased inward forces on the developing jaws. Overall, the focus is on parents trying to get in 'one more mouthful' and it promotes disengagement with the food or more mindless eating.

With BLW, the focus is on self-feeding. Babies control what they eat, how much they eat and how quickly they eat and reduce milk feeds. Parents or caregivers offer a variety of appropriate, grabbable foods in the form of sticks or strips, or food with a 'handle' – such as a lamb chop. Children get to explore different varieties, shapes, tastes, textures, and colours. Water is offered in a small open cup, and use of cutlery is delayed. Babies get to learn about different tastes and textures and experience shared mealtimes with the family. They also learn from their protective reflex of gagging how to chew properly, not to overfill their mouth, and not to push food too far back in the mouth.

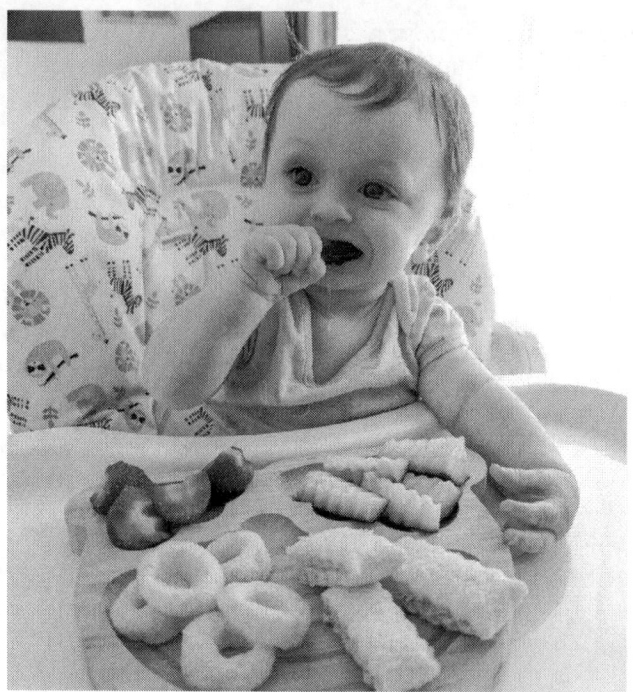

Parent photo used with consent

From six months, coinciding with when babies are able to sit upright, they will pick food up, take it to their mouth, and chew. They are naturally curious and eager to explore, mimic, and learn through observation. It helps them mature their gross and fine motor control, hand-eye coordination, and appetite control. Additional evidence suggests that it is feasible for most babies to enjoy a greater variety of foods which may potentially prevent obesity.

At the 2017 Academy of Applied Myofunctional Sciences Meeting in Chicago, Dr Christian Guilleminault suggested that when children had problems with sucking and swallowing earlier in life (for example, due to prematurity or tongue-ties), the introduction of foods requiring chewing would be a good opportunity for catch-up in muscle development and a reduction in the risk of developing sleep apnoea later in life.

Like many other airway-focused dentists, I see BLW as a great opportunity to offer this catch-up functional stimulation.

Most of this information, advice, practical tips, and the references can be found in Dr Rapley's book, which I highly recommend to any new parent to help them decide regarding introduction of solids.

Whatever parents decide, it is important not to transition too slowly to increased textures. 'Feeding is truly a developmental process, just like learning to crawl, walk, run. We would never do anything to keep a child from crawling,' speech and feeding therapist and author of the book *Raising a*

Healthy Eater: A Stage-By-Stage Guide to Setting Your Child on the Path to Adventurous Eating Melanie Potock says, 'Let's not do anything that would stall them in the development of eating.'

Pouch foods and sippy cups are other by-products of our busier, modern lives. They are aimed to offer greater convenience and reduced mess. Sippy cups are not a normal developmental stage a child has to pass through to open-cup drinking. Overuse of both may promote improper oral muscle and mouth development.

Despite seeming to offer the perfect combination of healthiness, the New York Times Article 'Rethinking Food Pouches' offers warnings by various experts of their impact on the environment, long-term dietary habits, and children's oral function.[25]

It highlights that excessive use may fail to challenge children at a critical stage of feeding and oral development – where chewing and swallowing also help with speech development and multi-sensory experiences to develop a palate for a wide range of foods later.

The ABC News article 'Are We Raising "Generation Suck" Who Drink Food with No Need for Chewing?' also highlights – among other problems – that abnormal oral function can hinder proper jaw development, speech development, and sensory literacy.[26]

The occasional pouch or sippy cup for convenience and less mess is not likely to create a big problem or stall feeding or speech development, but I agree that despite the increasing array and blends of organic foods with great nutritional value, the overuse of these pouch foods interferes with normal development.

Overall, I see children who prefer soft foods like pasta, cereal, and bread, and who would prefer mince or a burger over a nice cut of steak. As parents, we can all afford to rethink how we are obtaining our nutrition and whether we can help our children develop their muscles better.

In general, when mess is a concern, a straw cup may offer a better alternative than a sippy cup as it interferes less with normal tongue posture and the maturation of a normal swallow – with the tongue moving upward and back as opposed to thrusting forward.

For more information on normal feeding and oral development in the earliest years of life, I recommend *Feed Your Baby and Toddler Right: Early eating and drinking skills encourage the best development*. It is a good reference on what to expect at every feeding milestone so you can check your child's progress. It offers info on breastfeeding, spoon feeding, open cup and straw drinking, and ideal toys for mouthing to help a child bite, chew and explore, and prepare for eating, drinking, and speaking.

NORMAL CHEWING AND SWALLOWING

By six to seven months, we want to see a baby taking bites of food as opposed to sucking. They should be able to chew on small lumps of food – even without teeth – and should be able to move their tongue towards food in the sides of the mouth.

The digestive process starts in the mouth with good chewing and swallowing. Food needs to be broken down properly with good chewing and mixed with saliva to allow digestive enzymes to break down carbohydrates and other complex molecules.

By the age of 11 to 12 months we want to see a baby transition to a more mature swallow. The tongue helps collect the food and brings it to the centre of the tongue for swallowing. This tip of the tongue should lift to the area behind the front teeth.

If a child is using a lot of pacifiers, bottles, and sippy cups, is always spoon-fed foods that don't require chewing, has a tongue-tie, or has chronic open mouth posture, they may retain an infantile or tongue thrust swallow. This is a very inefficient way to swallow that is associated with excessive facial muscle use during swallowing, which impacts facial and dental development and the stability of orthodontic treatment results.

Case Study: 13-month-old with tongue tie and history of feeding issues

A 13-month-old patient was referred to me for a tongue-tie assessment. Her mum had no functional concerns about her daughter but wanted to see if a tongue-tie release should be performed to prevent future problems. Mom revealed a history of breastfeeding problems, including poor latch and pain, so she transitioned to formula to help her overcome the challenges when the baby was six weeks old.

I noted a severe restriction of tongue mobility. The mom also reported excessive drooling, heavy mouth breathing, and effortful breathing during sleep. She was a restless and hot sleeper, with her hair often soaked and matted on her face. I referred the patient for a speech and feeding assessment and the therapist noted that the patient's tongue could not move laterally or to the side. Therapy was commenced to strengthen her oral motor skills to support the success of the tongue-tie release.

At 16 months of age, the tongue-tie release was performed. Within one week, her mom reported that her child was saying more words, pronunciation was better, drooling had decreased, her tongue was able to move side to side while eating, and nasal breathing had replaced the effortful breathing of before, including less tossing and turning in her sleep.

This case demonstrates that when we improve muscle function with chewing, swallowing, and speech, there are often knock-on impacts on sleep and the airway. It makes total sense that these muscles serve so many common functions that there would be multiple impacts on a child's development.

It also demonstrates that parents sometimes may not be aware what is normal – in this case, mum didn't realise there was dysfunctional feeding. She also stated her daughter was a good sleeper, but there were signs of snoring, excessive sweating, and restlessness that indicated a risk of obstructive breathing, increased work of breathing, and a possibility of unrestorative sleep.

Unfortunately, it is too easy for problems to slip through the cracks or to get conflicting information. But when problems are properly addressed, there is a positive impact for the whole family.

Furthermore, when mum had her next baby and there were feeding problems despite an initial tongue-tie snip in hospital, mum knew to come straight to us to get the tongue-tie assessed and further managed. This allowed her to have a less stressful feeding experience the second time around.

CHEW ON THIS

Many children are not stimulating their chewing muscles optimally and have a deficit in muscle function. They may have been bottle fed or stuck in the suck phase with overly processed baby foods. Many children prefer softer foods like rice, pasta, minced meat, hamburgers, and sausages over a chewy piece of steak. These days it is common for children to have their fruits like apples cut up, or crusts cut off their sandwiches.

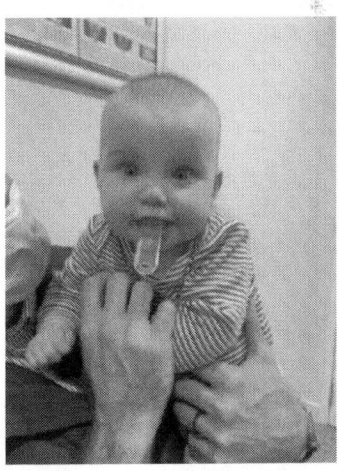

Used with parental consent

The Myo Munchee appliance is an important tool that can be used to offer an opportunity to catch up on closed mouth chewing practice. Children place it in their mouth and chew with their lips closed, most usually building up to two ten-minute periods per day. The main objectives of this activity are to:

- promote good lip seal
- encourage closed mouth chewing
- stimulate the chewing muscles evenly on both sides
- promote nasal breathing
- promote a more normal swallow – helps prevent forward thrusting of the tongue
- reduce inward pressures of the lip and cheek muscles during swallowing
- introduce more normal sensory input in children with sucking or other oral habits

They can also be a very good substitute for pacifiers that will not interfere with the tongue posture and can instead help re-establish lip seal and jaw closure.

The appliance can typically be introduced from the age of two years old, and I use them often as a tool to promote more normal function whilst waiting for children to become old enough to engage with myofunctional therapy. More recently the Myo Munchee company has introduced a version for babies called Bebe Munchee, which can be offered to babies under supervision from six months when they are able to sit up and grasp it.

I like the fact that it can efficiently retrain so many normal patterns at the same time when good compliance to regular use can be achieved. I suggest consulting with a dentist or myofunctional therapist prior to using one to get a baseline of dysfunction, and for more individualized recommendations on how to incorporate them in the total plan to restore more normal function.

Remember: the way our muscles work in the earliest years influences the way the jaws and facial structures grow. We've already seen how mouth breathing, breastfeeding, sucking habits, chewing, and swallowing can impact jaw and airway development.

Now, we will move onto the next chapter, where I will discuss how restricted tongue mobility and tongue-ties are further pieces of the puzzle to be aware of.

5

TONGUE-TIES

Widespread awareness of tongue-ties has been increasing in recent years, but it can be a source of confusion for parents with many conflicting professional opinions and polarizing debate on the topic.

A tongue-tie refers to when the attachment between the undersurface of the tongue is abnormally short or tight and restricts normal tongue mobility.

This can impact the tongue during sucking, swallowing, chewing, speech, and breathing, especially during sleep. In children, this impacts the way their palate and other facial structures grow.

Unfortunately, despite the impact on very critical functions, most of us health care professionals receive zero to minimal information in our training on tongue-ties or what normal tongue function looks like.

Even as a dentist, or so-called "physician of the mouth," I was taught nothing about tongue-ties in dental school. Nor was I taught anything about the role of the tongue in breastfeeding, palate development, and keeping the throat or upper airway open during sleep.

The field of tongue-tie research is relatively new, and there has been an explosion of published research and new knowledge on tongue-ties and their impact in the last decade.[1] Whilst there is some general awareness that tongue-ties have a role in breastfeeding challenges, there is now growing evidence to suggest that they are also linked to the development of breathing disturbances during sleep in childhood when they are not addressed in infancy. Despite this information coming to light, there remains a lag in its dissemination into educational institutions and clinical practices.

Tongue-tie diagnosis is not a fad. The need for more education and attention devoted to the topic has grown greater along with the increase in evidence. This chapter is about equipping you with the knowledge to know which problems to look out for so that you can better advocate for your child.

Problems that may be associated with tongue-ties include:

- infant feeding challenges
- speech delays and articulation problems
- chewing difficulties or fussy feeding
- mouth breathing, snoring, or teeth grinding
- poor oral rest posture and swallowing patterns
- abnormal palate and facial development
- the development of obstructive breathing during sleep
- increased neck and shoulder tension
- some migraines, tension, or other headaches

TONGUE-TIES AND BREASTFEEDING

Although I am involved in tongue-tie release from infancy to adulthood, my interest in tongue-tie management was first prompted by wanting to help more mothers and babies breastfeed for all the reasons discussed in the last chapter. I understood the main reasons for premature weaning from the breast are poor latching, pain, and the perception of low milk supply. Tongue-ties could be a potential contributor to each of these yet were often overlooked. I wanted to be part of the solution.

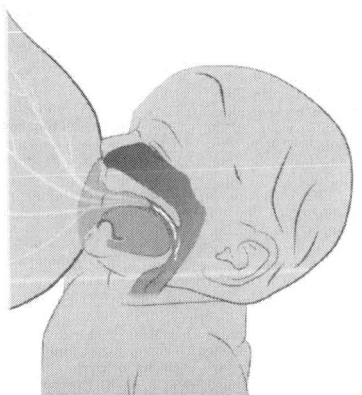
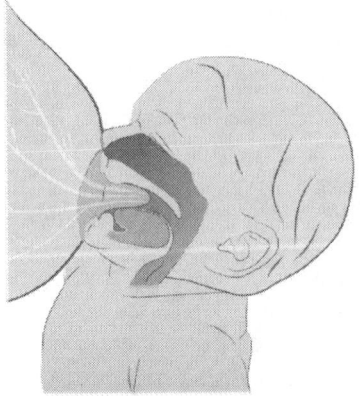

Normal Tongue Position   **Tongue Tie or Ankyloglossia**

In the last chapter, I highlighted how efficient transfer of milk from the breast is achieved with good tongue suction and the creation of an intra-oral vacuum. When mobility is restricted and the tongue is not free to elevate properly, a baby may compensate with overuse of their lips and cheeks. They may have a shallow latch and tend to slide or "gum" on the nipple. This can be associated with misshapen or blanched nipples, nipple trauma, and pain.

Other times, poor tongue suction is linked to inefficient transfer of milk and may manifest as symptoms such as the perception of low milk supply, poor drainage, blocked ducts and mastitis, or poor weight gain.

Reduced tongue mobility makes breastfeeding more effortful, and these babies may have prolonged feeds or fall asleep easily while feeding. Some may become increasingly frustrated, pulling on and off the breast during feeds.

These problems may not become obvious until after the first few months of breastfeeding, when milk production is less hormonally driven and linked closer to "demand," or how effectively an infant is transferring milk from the breast.

It's still a daily occurrence for me to see families struggling with these issues whose infants had their tongue-ties dismissed by numerous professionals, from paediatricians to lactation consultants. When they come to us, they are in a state of disappointment and are feeling let down by the system. Experiencing the improvements that come with intervention can sometimes relieve stress, anxiety, exhaustion, and guilt, and can also have a positive ripple effect on the rest of the family. It's key to understand that there is no one profession that has better training in this area when you are having problems – it's more important to find out who has most experience managing tongue-ties in infancy.

The prevalence of tongue-ties is reported to be in the range of 3-10% in various studies, but this usually only accounts for the obvious or visible anterior tongue-ties that attach all the way to the tip of the tongue.

Other times, tongue-ties are not as easy to identify, as they may only restrict the elevation of the middle to back portion of the tongue. These "posterior tongue-ties" are easily missed by health professionals who are not trained to lift the tongue to examine or palpate for these, or mistakenly think there is no problem because the tongue can extend forward.

Posterior tongue-ties can also be called "mild ties" based on their less obvious visual appearance. This is deceiving because they can still contribute to significant dysfunction and problems for both infants and mothers, including those affecting tongue suction and proper transfer of milk as well as the co-ordination of sucking and swallowing. Recent studies by ENT surgeon Dr Bobby Ghaheri have highlighted that surgery to address posterior tongue-ties can improve subjective measures such as reduction of pain, mother's confidence, and experience in feeding, and can also lead to reduced symptoms of reflux and even objective measures of sucking in bottle fed babies.[2-4]

For instance, both photos below illustrate tongue-ties that were contributing to feeding problems that were resolved with intervention.

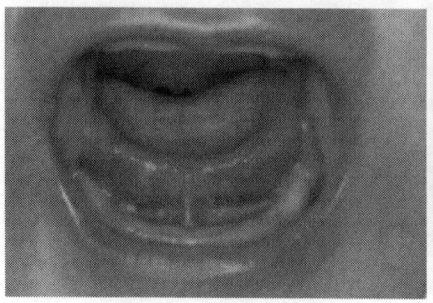 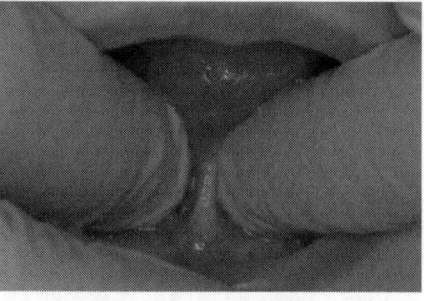

Anterior Tongue-Tie   **Posterior Tongue-Tie**

One of the difficulties around tongue-tie diagnosis is the lack of direct correlation between visual appearance and the degree of dysfunction or symptoms experienced. Many babies can adopt compensations – like overusing their other muscles to extract milk – while not developing the proper tongue suction that is the foundation for optimal breathing as they get older.

Tongue-tie diagnosis will depend on a combination of ALL of the following:

1. Infant and maternal symptoms
2. Feeding assessment with a lactation consultant or feeding therapist
3. Visual and physical assessment

Symptoms are a very important criteria in determining whether intervention should be considered. They can be broadly divided into those experienced by the infant and mother.

Infant symptoms:

- Shallow or unsustained latch (sliding off the nipple)
- Gumming, chewing, or clamping at the nipple
- Poor seal, clicking or smacking sounds
- Gulping of air
- Excess gas, colic, reflux, or vomiting
- Short, frequent feeds, or falls asleep at the breast easily
- Poor weight gain and failure to thrive
- Pulling on and off in frustration
- Snoring, congestion, or abnormal breathing
- Unable to hold a pacifier

Maternal symptoms:

- Creasing or blanching of nipples after feeding; lipstick-shaped nipple
- Blanching of the nipples
- Pain on latch or during feeding
- Cracking, bruising, blistering, or bleeding of the nipples
- Poor drainage, blocked ducts, or mastitis
- Perceived low milk supply
- Nipple infection or thrush
- Maternal guilt, exhaustion, or depression
- Premature weaning and change in the infant-mother relationship

As a dentist, I am not trained to assess the latch of feeding, but there are some visual clues in the mouth that indicate to me that things are not functioning well. These may present even in the absence of concerns with pain or weight gain.

Visual clues of oral dysfunction:

- Lip callousing or lip blisters
- Two toned lips
- Open mouth posture at rest
- Minimal lift of the tongue during crying
- Cupping or bowling of the tongue
- A heart shaped indent or forking of the tip of the tongue
- Milk remnant or white coating on the mid to back of the tongue

A professional well-trained on the implications of tongue-tie, lip-tie, and normal oral function will take all the above factors into consideration.

WHAT ABOUT LIP-TIES?

A lip-tie refers to when the attachment of the upper lip to the upper gum – where we expect the teeth to erupt in the future – is particularly tight and restricts upper lip mobility. This can be a barrier to establishing a good seal of the lips around the breast seen in an optimal latch. It can also contribute to excessive intake of air and reflux-like symptoms.

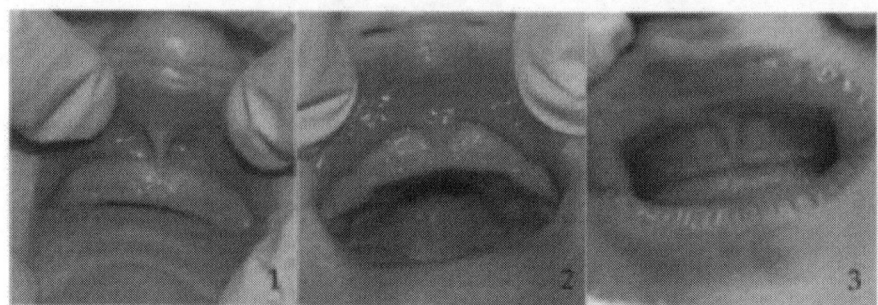

Supplied and used with permission by Dr Chloe Santa Maria, Stanford Department of Otolaryngology, Head and Neck Surgery

Researchers at Stanford photographed 100 babies to determine what was normal with lip ties.[5] They proposed a three-category classification system based on the level of attachment. They found that 80% of babies had a Grade 2 attachment (shown in the middle image), therefore making it common to have a fleshy attachment. It reinforces parents need not be immediately alarmed if they see this attachment if there are no problems.

A common concern for parents is whether lip ties will contribute to a gap between the front teeth. In the absence of functional issues or significant restriction of upper lip mobility, release is not usually recommended for this reason in babies since a gap cannot be predicted to occur. As the jaw grows, the attachment may relatively recede away from the teeth area and may not be a problem. In addition, a space between the baby teeth is completely normal to help maintain space for the larger adult teeth to fit. It is just as simple to release later if the problem with a gap between the adult teeth eventuates.

TONGUE-TIES, LIP TIES, AND REFLUX-LIKE SYMPTOMS

When a tongue-tie is not addressed early, it can lead to early weaning from the breast and the introduction of bottle feeding. A common misconception is that tongue-ties do not cause problems for bottle-fed babies. It is true that bottle feeding requires less effort to extract milk, which means that babies with tongue-ties may latch and feed more easily on a bottle. However, tongue-ties and lip-ties can often be a hidden cause of reflux-like symptoms in both breastfed and bottle-fed babies.

Acid reflux is a condition where the contents of the stomach are spit up shortly after feeding. Symptoms include:

- stomach distension or a hard belly
- unable to sleep lying down for long periods
- constant pain, crying or irritability

- prefer to be held upright
- waking congested in the morning
- belching, vomiting or excessive gas

When a child has a poor latch or seal, they may gulp excessive amounts of air. As this fills a baby's tummy, it can cause stomach distension and discomfort, and symptoms similar to acid reflux. The problem can be more accurately described as aerophagia or air-induced reflux, and acid reflux medications will not make a difference.

When paediatricians and medical practitioners do not take a breastfeeding history, it can lead to improper use of acid reflux medications primarily used in adults. The safety and effectiveness have not been properly validated for use in children. In fact, research links the use of these medications during infancy with increased risk of bone fractures later in childhood.[6]

On the other hand, there are now a handful of studies supporting a reduction in reflux-like symptoms in babies who had tongue and/or lip tie release.[2-4,7-10] Oral and Maxillofacial Surgeon Dr Scott Siegel published a retrospective review of 1,000 babies he performed tongue- and/or lip-tie surgery on.[7] These babies all had feeding problems and were also taking H2 Blockers or Proton Pump Inhibitors to manage reflux-like symptoms. He found that 52% had reversal of symptoms to the point they no longer required medication. A further 19% had post-surgical improvement in symptoms but were unable to be successfully weaned of medications.

Many mothers with a diagnosis of silent reflux spend lots of money trying various bottles, formulas, thickeners, colic mixtures, and reflux medications to help get a more comfortable baby. When none of these options work, parents are frequently assured their baby will grow out of it. This rarely offers any consolation for parents watching their baby suffer and feeling like they are neglecting their other children.

It makes complete sense to ask about how an infant is feeding before prescribing reflux medications to them. If there has been a history of breastfeeding challenges, it would be wise to seek a specially trained person to rule out lip- and tongue-ties as a contributor.

Case Study: 6-week-old infant with posterior tongue tie and reflux-like symptoms

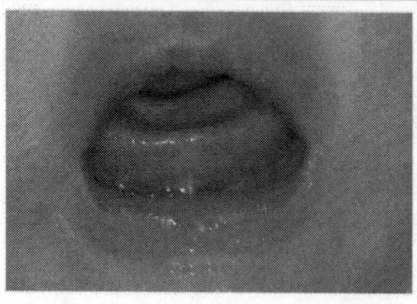 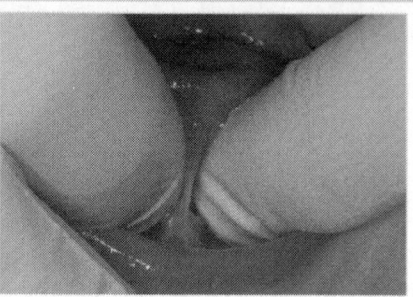

A six-week-old infant had a tongue-tie identified at birth. Mum had decided she was not going to breastfeed following a stressful feeding journey with her first baby relating to delayed identification of a tongue-tie. The paediatrician advised that tongue-tie release would not be required if they were not breastfeeding. The patient's parents sought a second opinion with me. At the time of the initial consult, the history included reflux-like symptoms, vomiting, gas, leakage during feedings, and more. A tongue-tie was confirmed so they continued with a release.

Three weeks after the tongue-tie release, the parents were able to cease reflux medications without negative impact. The baby's nasal congestion was completely gone, his gas symptoms were lessened, he slept better, and he proved to be a much happier baby all around.

The lack of clarity in relation to tongue-tie assessment and management was evident in the fact that the baby was prescribed reflux medications without consideration of poor latch and excessive swallowing of air. The baby had continual symptoms and discomfort which had an impact on the entire family. The mum was broken by the time she came to us. During her initial appointments, she was tearful and despondent. But by the time we saw her again, three weeks post-release, she was a different person. The weight had been lifted off her shoulders and she was very much more relaxed and able to smile again because of the improvements in her child.

It makes me wonder: what would have happened if there had been early identification and intervention of a tongue-tie with her first child? Could she have been more open to enjoying a breastfeeding relationship with this baby?

Babies learn to co-ordinate their sucking and swallowing in utero and releasing these tongue-ties is not going to guarantee normal function any more than taking a cast off an arm is going to automatically change function. Be aware a tongue-tie release does not necessarily result in a quick fix.

In general, the younger the infant, the better the chance of getting a good feeding outcome. An older infant will have developed more compensations that will be difficult to alter.

Support from a lactation consultant before and after the procedure to optimize latch and positioning, provide oral exercises to stimulate further tongue movement, and retrain suck patterns is helpful. Light physical therapy with a trained osteopath or craniosacral therapist to gently relax muscles that have been compensating for tongue restrictions, or to relax strains, compressions, and any nerve impingements that have been created through the in-utero or birth process is beneficial to promote optimal tongue function.

The primary objective of tongue-tie release is to improve mobility and facilitate better feeding during infancy. It is very realistic to expect that there will be some degree of persistent dysfunction that comes with altered patterns established well before birth, and it does not guarantee children can avoid future issues with speech, orthodontics, and sleep. As children get older, most will benefit from ongoing review and optimization of muscle function through feeding or myofunctional therapy.

TONGUE-TIES WITH FEEDING AND SPEECH CONCERNS

When tongue-ties are not addressed during infancy, the next functional problems that parents bring their children to see me with are issues with speech and feeding on solids.

In terms of speech development, speech issues can be related to speech delay or misarticulation problems. We now know that a free tongue is important to allow movement for speech perception. The tip makes tiny movements which provide sensory input to help distinguish between different sounds. Prolonged pacifier use or a tongue-tie may be implicated in speech delay.

Misarticulation may be related to lowered resting tongue posture and tongue thrust and poor co-ordination of the tongue tip to elevate the tongue to reach the roof of the mouth, behind the upper front teeth. Myofunctional therapy to help train more normal resting posture of the tongue-tie can often improve articulation even before release is performed.

Case Study: 4-year-old with tongue tie and concerns with speech and teeth grinding

We had a four-year-old patient in for speech and sleep concerns. This child's kindergarten teacher had suggested the patient see a speech pathologist due to concerns with articulation. His osteopath noted the classic heart-shape on the tip of his tongue and encouraged his family to seek a tongue-tie assessment with us. His parents were concerned about his articulation, their difficulty understanding him, his teeth grinding at night, and his restless sleeping.

We confirmed the presence of a tongue-tie and commenced myofunctional therapy to help restore normal tongue rest posture and tone in preparation for tongue-tie release. Great improvements were made in speech and the family was offered the option of delaying the surgery.

The observations made during his therapy with tongue exercises were that his articulation improved drastically (as commented by his teacher and family members who didn't see him regularly). At the start of the year, his parents made the decision to proceed with tongue-tie surgery to free up his tongue and give him the best opportunity to be confident at school.

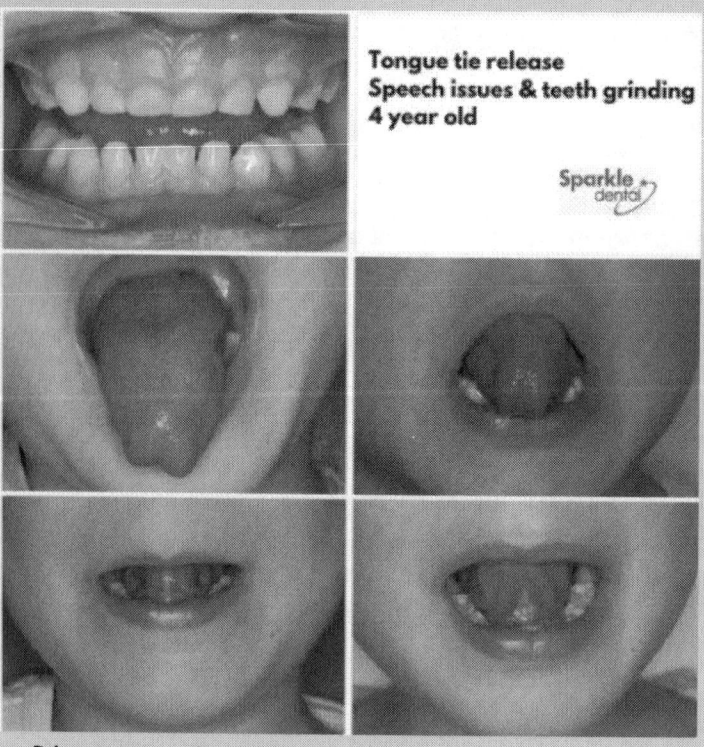

Tongue tie release
Speech issues & teeth grinding
4 year old

Sparkle dental

Prior to tongue-tie surgery   One week post-surgery

At two months post-surgery, his parents reported increased confidence, reading aloud more, talking more, use of bigger words, no teeth grinding during sleep, less restlessness, and sleeping a lot longer.

Incidentally, his osteopath has found that his feet are now straight (not turned in), and he no longer has problems with hip alignment. These types of postural improvements are commonly reported to us as well and can be linked to fascia – which will be mentioned later.

TONGUE-TIES, NARROW PALATES, AND POOR BREATHING

A child with a tongue-tie may still be able to breastfeed, speak, chew, and swallow without perceived problems. However, if the tongue's mobility is restricted, other muscles of the lips, cheeks, jaw, and even neck will be recruited in compensation. The ultimate problem is that the tongue does not develop sufficient tone to naturally rest in the roof of the mouth and properly fulfil its important role as a upper airway dilator muscle to keep the throat or upper airway open during sleep. This explains why a growing number of studies are now demonstrating an association between untreated tongue-ties and narrow palates, and the development of snoring and obstructive breathing in children.[10-18]

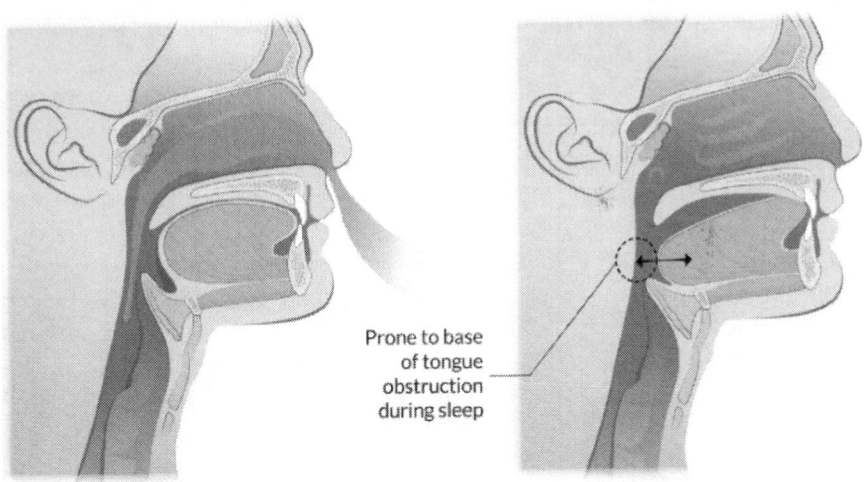

Prone to base
of tongue
obstruction
during sleep

Normal Tongue Posture

**Posterior Tongue Tie
Or Low Tongue Posture**

When the tongue lacks proper tone and can't elevate and suction to the roof of the mouth, it does not provide the proper seal with the soft palate to block off oral breathing. A person is more likely to become a mouth breather. Air does not flow as smoothly, and there is increased risk of airway collapse with increased efforts to breathe in to ensure air flows from the nose into the lungs. The back of the tongue is disused and becomes flaccid and is more likely to fall back and obstruct the airway during sleep.

A child or young adult is more likely to present with teeth grinding or Upper Airways Resistance Syndrome (UARS) – a precursor to OSA. The teeth grinding is a compensation to help recruit the jaw muscles to increase tone and function to reinstate and open airway. Stomach sleeping or restlessness can be other red flags that the base of the tongue is a risk factor in disturbed sleep breathing.

This is another important reason why we need to pay attention to the more "hidden" posterior tongue-tie that limits elevation of the back of the tongue.

The rationale for considering release is to improve tongue mobility and facilitate myofunctional therapy. You will find out more about this important intervention in Chapter 10.

It is gaining traction as a conservative option for people to restore nasal breathing and improve snoring and obstructive sleep apnoea. On average it can reduce OSA by 50% in adults and 62% in children.[19] These percentages could be improved further by ensuring there is enough space in the palate for the tongue to work well, and secondly by ensuring the tongue is not restricted. Tongue-tie release can therefore be considered a way to help make therapy more effective.

The myofunctional therapy process is begun prior to tongue-tie release and offers optimal benefits from the procedure. This allows practice and familiarity with exercises that may be continued immediately post release to interfere with the normal process of reattachment. It is common for patients to experience better breathing and sleep, clearer speech, or less choking on tablets or food with therapy even before tongue-tie release.

Exercises are continued after release to strengthen the back half of the tongue after years of disuse.

An ideal outcome for tongue-tie release is to achieve complete tongue-to-palate suction, closed mouth nasal breathing, and improved sleep. Often, palate expansion (expanded more in Chapter 9) will be necessary prior to improving space for the tongue to function and seal to the palate at rest properly.

TONGUE-TIES AND POSTURAL ISSUES

Another common consequence of restricted tongue mobility I tend to see manifest later in life is chronic head, neck, and shoulder tension.

The most common compensation pattern I see there is excess recruitment of the neck and shoulder muscles to move the tongue. This chronic overuse during normal function can lead to the development of hypersensitive knots in the tight bands of neck muscles called trigger points. These can cause myofascial or referred pain to the head. Patients may complain of regular headaches that they perceive as originating from their neck or that coincide with when their neck feels tight. These headaches referred from the neck are called cervicogenic headaches. Often these patients will go to regular chiropractic or physio appointments for relief, but reductions in tension do not hold.

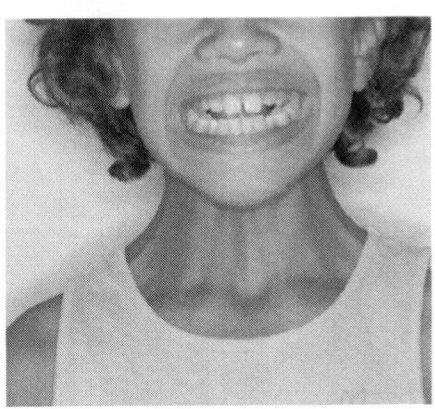

Myofunctional therapy and tongue-tie release may be an option to restore normal tongue mobility and function to alleviate these symptoms. ENT surgeon Dr Soroush Zaghi is responsible for pioneering work to advance our understanding in this area. He has published a case series of 348 patients who had myofunctional therapy for reasons including mouth breathing, snoring, clenching, and myofascial tension, and who he also performed tongue-tie surgery on to facilitate better therapy.[20]

He found an overall satisfaction rate of 91% with improvements in mouth breathing (78.4%), snoring (72.9%), clenching (91%) and myofascial tension (77.5%). Patients who didn't have improvements tended to be those with limited space due to improper jaw size and position.

A network of connective tissue called 'fascia' helps to explain the referred pain patterns and potential for improvements in body tension. It forms the framework of our body, surrounding and holding every organ, blood vessel, bone, nerve fibre, and muscle in place. The deep front-line fascia runs from the tongue through all our midline structures and into our toes. If there is a tongue-tie, the fascia within it will be tight and this will create tension and areas of restriction in areas far beyond the tongue.

I work closely with craniosacral therapists and other physical therapists for all tongue-tie releases to help release fascia in the rest of the body. Adult patients tend to report release of neck and shoulder tension, greater neck mobility, and less forward head posture after tongue-tie surgery in conjunction with myofunctional therapy. Some patients report greater ease in breathing, which may be linked to release of the fascial strains around the diaphragm, noted by manual therapists that we work closely with.

• • •

The take home message is that this tiny string under our tongue can play out with significant problems from infancy to adulthood, yet it is commonly overlooked. When the tongue has not functioned properly, the problems are compounded with poor structural development of the jaws, meaning more intervention will be required to eliminate compensations and restore normal functions.

At the same, whilst intervening in infancy can promote better function, children still need regular follow ups to make sure the mouth is working and growing properly as they get older.

The next chapter will help you identify the earliest warning signs that jaw development is off track.

SMALL JAWS AND CROOKED TEETH

In industrialized countries, crooked teeth are becoming more prevalent, and it's widely accepted that braces will be a necessity, and normal rite of passage for children as they enter their teenage years. But this does not have be the case.

Crooked teeth are one of the recognizable warning signs of poor jaw and airway development. However, current practice is often to wait until a child is 12 to begin treatment – when much of the facial and jaw structures are built and set. We introduced this topic in Chapter 2, but now I will go into how this should factor into your decisions regarding orthodontic treatment for your children. It's time to start connecting crooked teeth to poor jaw development, some degree of limitation of normal airflow, and sub-optimal breathing and sleep. This will impact each child to varying degrees, and we know some will fall short of their full potential.

In Chapter 2, we established that the shrinking jaws could be largely related to reduced functional stimulus of the muscles. This phenomenon reflects modern living, including a shift from paleolithic diets that required intense chewing to soft and overly processed diets in industrial times. This has coincided with a reduced duration of breastfeeding, increased use of pacifiers, and increased allergies and mouth breathing.

British orthodontist Dr Mike Mew describes how, as muscles have become weaker and the mouth more open, jaws are no longer growing wide and forward, but more vertical and backwards. He describes this phenomenon as "melting of the human face" – as if the face was made of candle wax and a flame was held before it. The upper jaw flattens, giving rise to flattened cheekbones, and the lower jaw starts melting down and back, resulting in longer faces and recessed chins. The reduced chin prominence can be linked to bags under the eyes and reduced support for the nasal cartilage, making the nose seem large and hooked. Not only do faces become less attractive, but this leads to reduced airways and space for the tongue.

In one of the most widely downloaded articles in the British Dental Journal from 2014, Dr Mew uses the term Craniofacial Dystrophy to describe how crooked teeth are only one symptom of a much larger problem.[1]

When the jaws don't grow well, there is a distortion of our entire cranial and facial skeleton. This disharmony can be linked to TMD or pain and dysfunction of our jaw, joint, and chewing muscles, or headaches. It is linked to ear, nose, and throat (ENT) problems like deviated septums, sinusitis, narrow nasal passages, middle ear infections, glue ear, and eustachian tube dysfunction. The upper jaw forms part of the orbits, and we are also seeing more research linking narrow palates with vision problems.[2]

Most critically, poor jaw growth is associated with reduced tongue space and constricted or pinched airways and the increasing prevalence of snoring and sleep disturbed breathing.

Impacted wisdom teeth make up another relatively new phenomenon which has only occurred in the last few hundred years. This is thought to be part of the same process. The wisdom teeth are the last teeth to erupt in the mouth, and due to the reduced chewing of hard foods and stimulation of jaw growth, there is less room for these teeth. In non-Westernised societies, there is virtually no incidence of impacted wisdom teeth.

In other words, crooked teeth, impacted wisdom teeth, jaw, joint, and muscle pain, dysfunction and snoring, and sleep apnoea all have the same root cause and can all be considered diseases of modern civilisation.

It is possible to tell a child is developing an orthodontic problem as early as when the baby teeth emerge. During this early period of rapid development, not only are the teeth and mouth affected, but children in this stage also have the highest need for restorative sleep, as their brains are rapidly growing and making lots of neural connections that form the basis for future learning.

If we wait until a child is 12 years old to address their orthodontic needs, the focus will be on straightening the teeth and adjusting the bite to jaws that are not properly grown or developed. All too often, healthy permanent teeth must be removed to alleviate dental crowding. Meanwhile, many of the contributing factors to poor facial development are disregarded. It is not uncommon, therefore, for teeth to relapse back to their original positions after orthodontic treatment, particularly when retainers are lost or forgotten.

There are some orthodontists who offer an early phase of orthodontics around the age of seven or eight years, using dental appliances to modify the growth of the jaws and help create more space for the permanent teeth. Both the American and Australian associations of orthodontists advise that children have an orthodontics assessment no later than the age of seven years. However, from a facial and airway perspective, this is still too late.

Paediatric dentist Dr Kevin Boyd coined the term 'Cranio–Facial–Respiratory Complex' (CFRC) to help stop people thinking about teeth and focus instead on the importance of the jaw and facial region for breathing. Dr Boyd suggests when it comes to optimising the CFRC, patients presenting at age seven can be considered 'geriatric.'

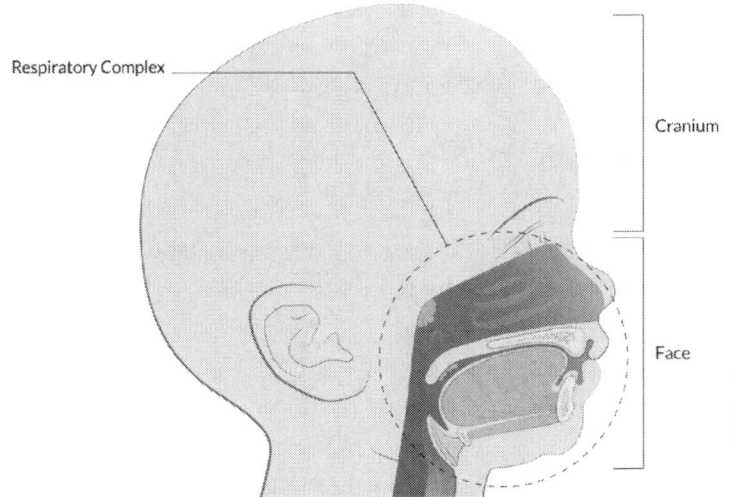

Quite often, the common orthodontic practice is to wait and delay intervention to straighten teeth until the jaws have stopped growing. Many parents are confused by this because they see the dental problem getting worse with time. But the bigger problem is summed up by this question: what impact does suboptimal airway development have on a child, and how will the future play out for them?

Dr Boyd likens delaying orthodontic treatment to telling a parent to wait until their four-year-old child is 10 years old before getting glasses for their shortsightedness because they will need a new pair each year until they are done growing. What experiences will that child miss out on in the six years between?

Intervening at a very young age – when there is a lot of growth potential remaining – also means addressing the soft tissue dysfunction or muscle imbalances to ensure lasting results. This may include introducing palate expansion when a child still has all their baby teeth in contrast to waiting until the first adult teeth come through.

These days, it is unusual to see a child with jaws that will naturally develop with room for the adult teeth.

These photos illustrate what is normal when a child has all their baby teeth.

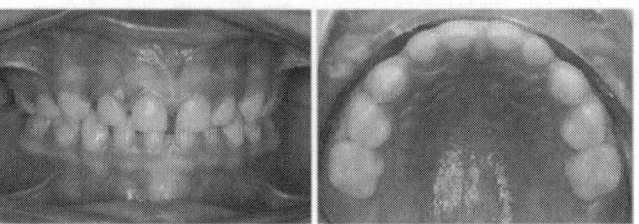

Ideal bite characteristics in children with baby teeth include:

- The top teeth and jaw fit over the lower teeth like a lid over a shoebox.
- The upper jaw is broad and U-shaped.
- There are gaps between the front baby teeth.
- The top front teeth only slightly overlap the bottom front teeth in the vertical and horizontal direction.

Deviations from the above can indicate that the tongue does not rest properly in the roof of the mouth and there is an imbalance of the orofacial muscles.

COMMON BITE PROBLEMS

These are some common bite issues that can be detected when children have baby teeth. What all these variations have in common is that the tongue is not providing adequate functional stimulation for the palate or upper jaw to develop; the lower jaw will also begin to suffer as a result.

Posterior Crossbite

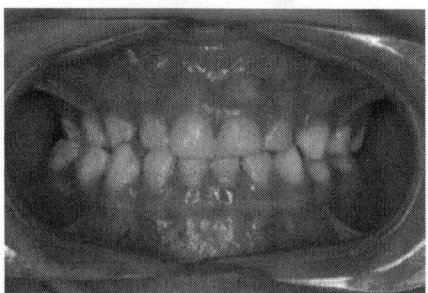

When the upper jaw is too narrow, a 'functional shift' of the lower jaw may occur. It swings to one side to achieve maximum contact between the upper and lower teeth. In this case, note the lack of spacing present between the front teeth, and how the midlines of the upper and lower teeth do not coincide. The former is a good indication the jaw is not growing enough to allow all the permanent teeth to fit into alignment. These crossbites are most commonly associated with pacifier and dummy use, and persistent dysfunctional swallowing even after their use is ceased.[3]

If this poor growth pattern is left unchecked, it can result in asymmetric facial growth with increasing deviation of the chin to one side. Research suggests that this type of orthodontic problem is associated with an increased risk in the poor development of jaw joints, as well as muscle pain and dysfunction in the long term.[4]

Anterior Crossbite

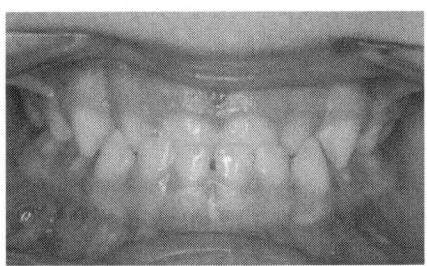

This type of problem is when the upper front teeth sit behind the lower front teeth, blocking the normal forward development of the upper jaw. Again, in this example, note the lack of spacing between the front teeth.

Anterior crossbite most commonly occurs in association with very low tongue posture. This is usually accompanied by either a tongue-tie or enlarged tonsils.[5-6] If there are enlarged tonsils within the throat, a child may habitually posture their jaw forward to help open their airway and this can exacerbate the problem.

When this is untreated and upper jaw growth is locked in or restrained, midface deficiency or a flat facial profile may result. As the child grows, their lower jaw becomes disproportionally prominent. Many people know this as an underbite or a class III jaw relationship.

This facial pattern often runs in families, with parents aware that surgery may be required to correct this problem once the jaws have stopped growing. However, if a child's upper jaw development can be optimized as early as possible, they will be less likely to need surgery in the future.

Deep Bite

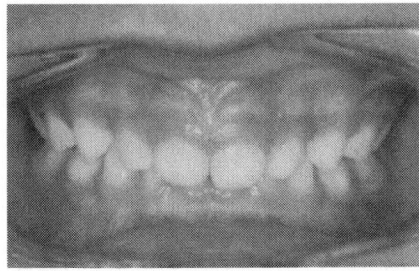

A deep bite refers to when the top front teeth vertically overlap the lower front teeth by more than two to three millimetres.

They are called 'traumatic deep bites' when there is complete vertical overlap, and the lower teeth impinge on the gum tissue behind the upper front teeth. It is my observation that these are commonly associated with lateral tongue thrusts. In this situation the back portion of the tongue often rests between the upper and lower teeth, including during sleep. This allows supra-eruption of the lower front teeth, creating a deepening of the bite.

Deep bites trap the lower jaw from developing or moving forward freely and are known to be associated with increased risk of jaw joint and muscle dysfunction.[7]

It is a common pattern for my adult patients diagnosed with obstructive sleep apnoea to have deep bites. I also find that these patients are more prone to wear on their front teeth, which can reflect the top jaw intermittently sliding forward during sleep to open the airway.

Anterior Open Bite

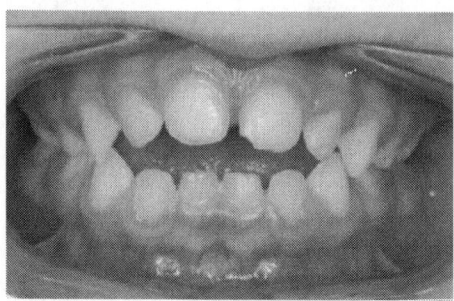

An open bite is associated with the use of pacifiers, thumb sucking, or tongue thrusts (or lowered tongue posture). This case was associated with prolonged pacifier sucking; the sucking forces of the cheeks resulted in inward pressures which narrowed the upper jaw. In compensation, the back teeth appear tilted inwards.

While open bites may close spontaneously once the sucking or poor postural habit is eliminated, incorrect resting posture and swallowing often persist.

Excess Dental Overjet

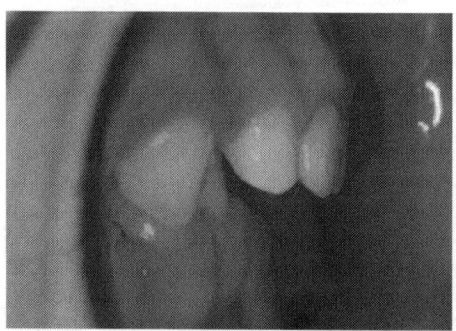

The situation where the horizontal overlap between the upper front teeth and lower front teeth is more than several millimetres is commonly referred to as "an overbite" by parents. This reflects some degree of underdevelopment of the lower jaw, which is a well-known risk factor for sleep disturbed breathing in both childhood and adulthood. Although it could be misconceived that the upper jaw is too protrusive, research suggests that it is more likely the upper jaw is also underdeveloped and retruded, and this is linked to a vertical growth pattern.[8]

Whereas upper jaw development is largely influenced by tongue posture and mode of breathing at rest, lower jaw development is a determined by proper functional stimulation during breastfeeding, chewing, and swallowing.

This degree of overjet, when it appears so early, will tend to worsen as time passes. It will become more difficult for the lips to seal easily, and the lower lip will get trapped between the teeth at rest, compounding the dysfunction.

These children are more likely to have dental trauma or accidents or be prone to bullying and self-esteem issues related to their teeth. In all these malocclusions or bite problems, there is some degree of underdevelopment of the palate: the template for lower jaw development.

Addressing constricted palates during the window of peak jaw development is essential if we want to break the continuous interaction of poor form and function and unlock the lower jaw so it may grow freely.

A MYOFUNCTIONAL APPROACH TO ORTHODONTICS

Traditional orthodontics focuses on utilizing a mechanical treatment approach to achieve straight teeth, despite the underlying muscle dysfunction or biological basis of the problem. Control is most often in the hands of the orthodontist who uses braces, palate expanders, or other devices that generate tooth movements and eliminate or minimize the need for co-operation.

In contrast, a myofunctional orthodontic approach focuses on addressing the muscle dysfunctions that contribute to crooked teeth. Straighter teeth become a secondary outcome. The timing to commence treatment is not related to whether permanent teeth are present but instead is based on intervening earlier when poor muscle habits are first identified. Placing the emphasis on achieving better muscle function and balance allows the jaws to develop more optimally and for the teeth to grow into the right place.

One of the key aspects of myofunctional orthodontics is exercises to promote proper tongue tone and posture, nasal breathing with good lip seal, and good swallowing through therapy. Sometimes myofunctional training appliances are used, which are soft, prefabricated appliances produced by different manufacturers, going by proprietary names such as Myobrace or Healthy Start. They are normally prescribed for one-hour-a-day wear and overnight wear.

The purpose of these appliances is to address the soft tissue dysfunctions contributing to poor facial development. There is usually a tongue tag or tongue shelf to help promote proper resting posture of the tongue. Children develop the lip tone and seal to keep it in their mouth and breathe through their nose. The appliances also encourage correct posturing of the lower jaw with tissue shields that help reduce overactivity of the facial muscles and the abnormal forces that act against normal facial development.

These appliances have been used for several decades and are highly compliance based. They are usually used in conjunction with exercises.

Up until a few years ago, I was deferring palate expansion until age six to eight years and would focus solely on restoring normal muscle function in even younger children. My rationale was that they are growing rapidly at this time so they have a lot of growth potential remaining that can be redirected if we can normalize muscle functions.

However, I now perceive that myofunctional orthodontics is often best combined with early palate expansion to optimize nasal breathing and make space for the tongue to function properly, as I have consistently seen the positive impact of palate expansion on children with breathing and sleep problems. My aim is to optimize sleep and breathing as early as I can to promote more optimal brain and facial development. Chapter 9 will cover palate expansion for children in greater detail.

Myofunctional orthodontics is time intensive and requires a massive shift in the way most orthodontic practices operate.

Orthodontist Dr Barry Raphael, who has shifted to this integrative approach in his practice, suggests "traditional orthodontics can be compared to bariatric surgery or cardiac bypass surgery where we are treating the symptoms of longstanding problems that have gone too far. Conversely, myofunctional orthodontics can be compared to healthy eating and living that will avoid such issues... Obviously the latter is preferable, though we know how difficult establishing healthy habits can be."

With the understanding that poor muscle habits are directly implicated in poor sleep, health outcomes, and a poor trajectory of facial development, it makes the re-establishment of continuous nasal breathing an important goal to pursue.

CROOKED TEETH, EXTRACTIONS, AND SLEEP DISORDERED BREATHING

The increase in dental professionals getting involved with managing sleep disordered breathing has brought with it an increase in debate and controversy surrounding the practice of extracting teeth to relieve dental crowding.

There has only ever been one research study by Dr Guilleminault and co-workers that compared objective sleep study data of children who presented with symptoms of OSA.[9] The researchers included 43 children with missing teeth (31 who had congenitally missing teeth, and 11 with orthodontic extractions), and 43 children matched for age, gender, and BMI but with enlarged adenoids and tonsils and no missing teeth.

They found that children with missing teeth tended to develop more symptoms at a later age, with higher AHI scores (more severe OSA) compared to those with enlarged adenoids and tonsils. Having missing teeth was linked to reduced jawbone and structural support of the airway, leading to increased collapsibility during sleep.

Despite the existence of this data, there is some resistance to the challenge to traditional orthodontic practice; people want to see even more evidence. It is unlikely there will ever be a black-and-white, universally accepted answer to the question of whether orthodontic extractions lead to OSA.

OSA is an end-stage breathing dysfunction that may take decades to develop, and it is costly and impractical to investigate with sleep studies on a large scale, let alone with adequate follow up.

What is indisputable is the fact that crooked teeth reflect underdeveloped jaws, and underdeveloped jaws are well-known risk factors for the development of obstructive breathing. They are linked to narrow nasal floors, increased resistance to nasal breathing, reduced tongue space, and reduced support for our collapsible tube of upper airway muscles.

There needs to be greater recognition that crooked teeth equates to airflow limitation.

At the time of writing this book, I have been involved in managing OSA for over a decade. I see the detrimental impact on health, energy, mood, cognitive function, and quality of life in my patients.

My interest is in optimizing jaw and airway development early to achieve a better trajectory of sleep, breathing and quality of life for people. If we are deciding whether to take out teeth to straighten them and/or alleviate crowding, we have already missed the boat.

Orthodontic extractions don't cause OSA. The underlying structural deficiency is the risk factor, and OSA is the very end stage of the continuum of breathing abnormalities and airway dysfunction. The question we need to be asking is this: how can we develop the jaws early in life to optimize airway, sleep, health, and wellness for life?

My journey with orthodontics began when I first understood that palate widening could help children breathe better. It made complete sense to me to develop the jaw properly so that the teeth would fit. We were taught in dental school that ages seven to eight was the optimal window to refer for orthodontic treatment if dental crowding was becoming apparent.

I was referring patients to the orthodontist, but they weren't doing anything. I would receive feedback that the orthodontist had assessed the situation and the patient was being placed on regular recall to observe their growth and treatment would be commenced once that was almost complete and stable.

Then, around the patient's age of twelve years, I would get another letter saying the child was ready for braces and asking if I could please remove two to four of their adult premolar teeth before their treatment commenced.

I tried to speak to a couple of the local orthodontists about doing palate expansion for patients, but it just wasn't an efficient option for them. They stated early treatment was unstable and prone to relapse. There was no interest in addressing the root causes of poor jaw development. Doing treatment in one round would be efficient, predictable, and avoid burnout. Achieving straight teeth as quickly as possible was their primary goal – a goal which didn't align with mine.

This prompted me to learn more and enroll in a two-year mini residency with Sydney orthodontist Dr Derek Mahony to learn more about interceptive and non-extraction orthodontics. Dr Mahony was ahead of the times in understanding the importance of proper jaw development for breathing and an early phase of treatment while the jaws were growing.

He was also well-sought after by parents for his reputation in avoiding extractions when multiple other orthodontists were recommending them. I was passionate about avoiding orthodontic extractions because I could see the problems in my adult patients years down the line when their lack of tongue space was exacerbated with retractive orthodontics. There was a relapse of results, teeth grinding, poor breathing and sleep, and jaw joint or muscle dysfunction. Some also had flattening of the facial profile.

This is one of the cases I completed when I started offering orthodontic treatment as a general dentist.

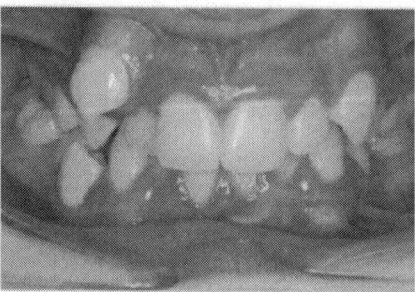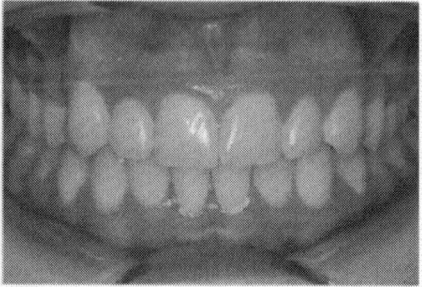

When we see this severity of crowding, we know that the tongue has not rested on the palate to stimulate proper development of the palate's width. The patient's parents reported chronic mouth breathing, snoring, restlessness during sleep, and bedwetting – all known red flags for obstructive breathing during sleep.

This child's family were told he required extraction of teeth to manage the crowding. He presented with dark circles under his eyes that indicated unrestorative sleep, and there were concerns with his concentration at school.

We aligned the teeth without any premolars extracted within 18 months. At the same time, his crossbite was corrected, and more oral volume for his tongue to rest and function properly was created. The patient and his family were happy with their choice not to remove teeth. It's a pleasure to see his eyes light up when he displays his broad post-treatment smile during his regular dental visits.

In combination with orthodontic treatment, I referred him to an ENT specialist who removed enlarged adenoids and turbinates. His breathing improved and the bedwetting ceased immediately.

This example reinforces the reality that professional opinions can vary. If advice has been given to take out structurally sound teeth before orthodontic treatment, it can be worth getting a second opinion to see if more space can be created to accommodate them before going ahead with extractions.

These days, I don't offer orthodontic treatment for children beyond the ages of seven to nine years. I am most passionate and focused on early intervention and am seeing children much earlier to help set up good habits and muscle patterns or offering early palate widening to prevent this situation from developing.

But the big question for children like this is: what is the lost potential from not addressing the breathing dysfunction earlier? Could this particular child have enjoyed school better if he'd been able to focus and concentrate easier?

Hopefully, if we intervene early to ensure children have the optimal functional patterns – including nasal breathing from birth – or offer some early interceptive orthodontics, development will be on a better track and treatment will be limited to minor aesthetic alignment.

Too often I see children who I wish I could have seen much earlier to guide growth and development in the right direction.

Let's explore some of the solutions to restore airway health in the following section to be able to advocate better for our child when needed.

PART III

PATHWAYS TO RESTORE AIRWAY HEALTH

7

SLEEP AND AIRWAY SCREENINGS

We've now discussed the importance of nasal breathing and restorative sleep for children and identified some of the developmental milestones where airway health can go off track. This next section is all about common treatment avenues that will lead to better airway structure and function for your child.

The first step is a screening to assess for sleep and airway problems and identify the need for further investigation. From here, you can move on to selecting potential targets for treatment and who will be part of your child's integrative team.

> The American Academic of Pediatrics' guidelines from 2012 suggest all children must be screened by health care professionals for snoring.[1]

However, this is not something that always occurs in practice. An Australian study found that general medical practioners enquired about a child's sleep only 11.4% of the time when they had a clinically significant sleep disturbance based on their "Sleep Disturbance Scale for Children" scores.[2] In addition, whilst 25% of children attending for "sick visits" at their GP had a clinically significant sleep disturbance, only 15.2% of those parents raised sleep concerns during their visit. This lack of follow up and concern leaves many children untreated.

A survey of over 400 medical schools in 12 countries found that the average amount of time spent on sleep education from respondents was two and a half hours, with an average of 17 minutes allocated to children's sleep.[3] This is despite sleep being a key pillar of healthy child development. **It's up to parents to be their child's best sleep advocate and raise concerns.**

Though we went over them briefly in Chapter 1, here's a refresher on the signs and symptoms that may suggest that a child is not getting the full benefits of restorative sleep or is at risk of breathing difficulties.

Night-time clues:

- Mouth breathing
- Snoring or audible breathing
- Gasping for air or pauses in breathing
- Neck hyperextension or sleeping in awkward positions including stomach sleeping
- Frequent tossing and turning
- Sweating
- Teeth grinding
- Bedwetting
- Frequent awakenings
- Nightmares or terrors

Day-time clues:

- Feeling unrefreshed on waking
- Headaches
- Tiredness or sleepiness during the day
- Hyperactivity
- Poor concentration or attention
- Behavioural concerns
- Prone to meltdowns or tantrums
- Defiance or aggressive behaviour
- Anxiety
- Difficulties with learning
- Poor school performance

Be aware that many of these symptoms can occur together without any snoring. This is because children can compensate to keep their airway open with open mouth breathing, sleeping with their head tilted back or on their stomachs, grinding their teeth, or tossing and turning to find a better position.

We want to see children breathing quietly, still and effortlessly (without building up a sweat), and through their nose to get the most restorative sleep and help with their daytime function.

> **If you recognise a problem with your child's breathing during sleep, arm yourself with photos or videos of any open mouth breathing, snoring, gasping, restlessness, or unusual sleep positions to support your concerns.**

If your child has symptoms of ADHD, ensure airway problems are fully investigated and managed before medicating them to avoid a misdiagnosis.

In Australia, your GP can help organize a referral to an Ear Nose and Throat (ENT) specialist or to a sleep specialist who can arrange a sleep study to investigate this further. Alternatively, airway focused dentists like myself are happy to discuss your concerns and screen children for airway and breathing disorders and help you navigate the road ahead. We can also organize direct referrals to an ENT. Referrals to a sleep physician or for a sleep study from a dentist will not attract a Medicare Rebate.

In 2017, the American Dental Association's House of Delegates adopted a policy statement called 'The Role of Dentistry in the Treatment of Sleep Related Breathing Disorders.'[4] It reinforced the dentists' important role both in screening for risks of sleep related breathing disorders and in identifying signs of deficient jaw development in children. It suggested that if a patient is at risk of obstructive breathing, then referral for both medical and dental evidence-based treatment may be appropriate to treat the breathing problem and/or develop a better airway and breathing pattern.

There are three key reasons why dental professionals have a central role in identifying at-risk children and coordinating care.

Firstly, we are largely a preventive care-based profession and see children on a regular six-month basis, often before their first GP visit. Whilst many paediatricians and general medical practitioners are busy taking care of diseases and illnesses, dentists can play a very important role in ensuring children at risk of future problems are directed to care at the earliest opportunity.

We update our patients' medical histories at every appointment, so adding a few extra questions about sleep symptoms is easy. We can be more alert to signs and symptoms of sleep breathing difficulties when we see those with medical risk factors such as obesity, allergies, asthma, gastroesophageal reflux disease (GERD), a history of prematurity or syndromes affecting the craniofacial features or neuromuscular disease, or a history of prematurity.

Secondly, there are many clues in the face and inside the mouth that give dentists an indication of a child who may be at risk of problems, and I'm going to walk you through the clues that I look for routinely in my patients further along in this chapter.

Thirdly, as some of the interventions that can address specific risk factors involve the mouth, more dental professionals are getting trained in this area. This can include palate widening, tongue-tie management, and myofunctional therapy.

A well-trained dentist will be able to act as the quarterback for your child's airway health and discuss various options and co-ordinate referral to other professionals for care.[5-8]

To find out whether a dentist is airway aware, you can ask the following questions:

- Do you regularly screen for airway and sleep and breathing problems in children?
- Do you ever refer children to an ENT for an airway assessment?
- Do you work with a myofunctional therapist to address mouth breathing?
- Do you offer or refer for orthodontic treatment for children before their adult teeth come through?
- Do you offer or refer for tongue tie release?

A team that is well versed in each of these areas will be able to help co-ordinate an integrative and collaborative approach.

WHAT AN AIRWAY-TRAINED DENTIST WILL LOOK FOR DURING THEIR ASSESSMENT

Forward head posture. When your child is standing and you view them from the side, is their ear vertically in line with their shoulders? If the ear is significantly ahead then this is considered forward head posture. It is most associated with low tongue posture and is thought to be a compensation pattern to keep an open airway. Like in CPR, the forward jaw thrust helps open the airway for better breathing. To maintain vision ahead, the neck and other muscles compensate, and this can lead to curvature of the cervical (neck) spine, neck pain, and a hunched upper back.

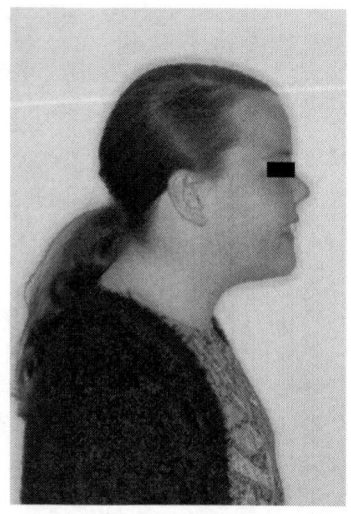

Venous pooling or allergic shiners. Do they have dark circles under their eyes that look like bruises? These may be a symptom of allergies and congestion in the nose, which increases blood flow in the area. The darkness is caused by the pooling of blood in the veins as it drains through a relatively tight space under the eyes. This problem can be compounded when the midface has not developed forward fully.

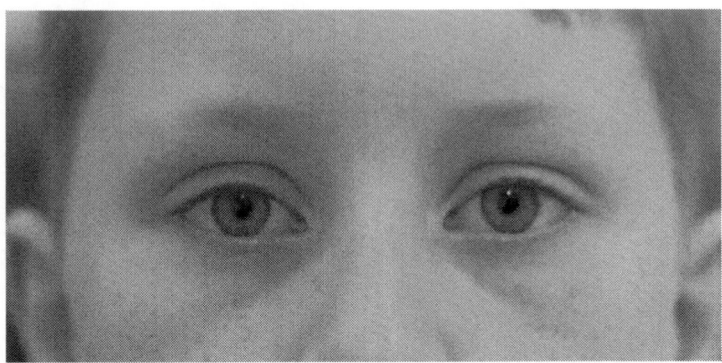

Open mouth, dry or chapped lips, or strain when closing lips together. These are all indications that a child has a pattern of mouth breathing. If they are not able to seal their lips together without strain, then we can be certain they spend a significant amount of the time with their mouth open during sleep when all the muscles have reduced tone.

Mentalis strain is the golf ball or dimpled appearance of the chin when the lips are sealed together. It indicates that the lips are not likely to seal during sleep. A recently published study in the Journal of the American Paediatric Dentistry found that it was number two out of 15 warning signs in the mouth that could predict a child had disturbed sleep breathing.[9]

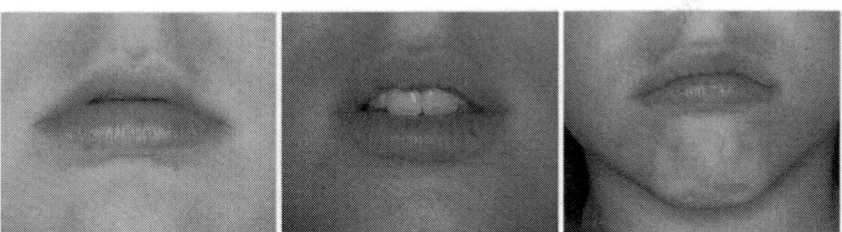

Their facial profile. Alterations in facial development include a long face/vertical growth pattern (also called adenoid facies), retruded lower jaw, midface deficiency, or relatively straight profile.[10,11]

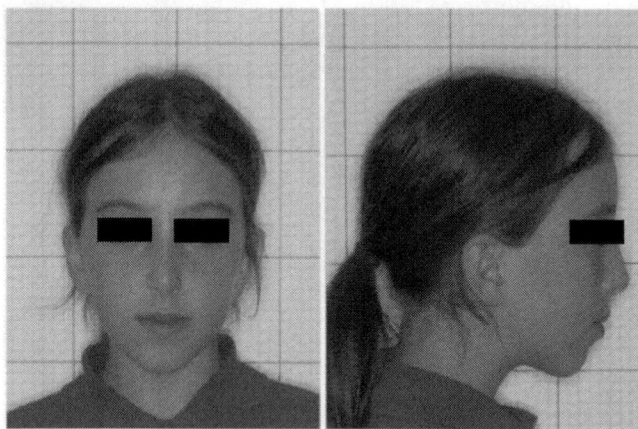

Vertical growth pattern or adenoid faces

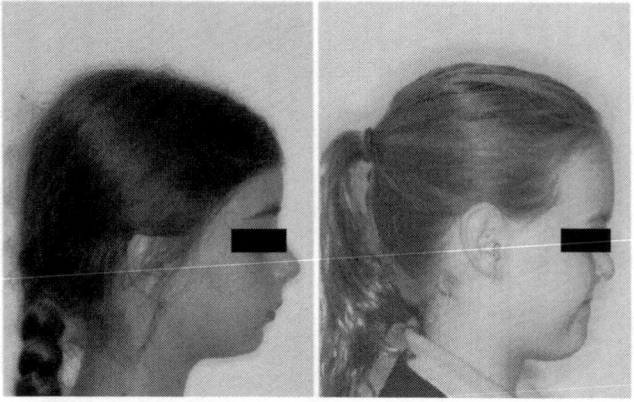

Receded lower jaw (left) and sunken or flat facial profile (right)

Gummy smiles. In general, we want the jaws to grow wide and forward. A gummy smile could be a subtle indicator that the upper jaw is growing in a more vertical direction with the lower jaw swinging down and back.

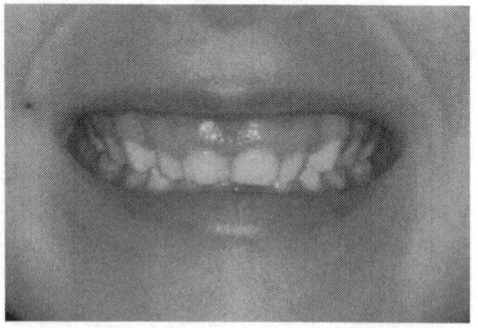

Sclera show. Whites being visible under the irises can be a subtle sign of lack of forward development of the upper jaw. This leads to reduced support of the orbits.

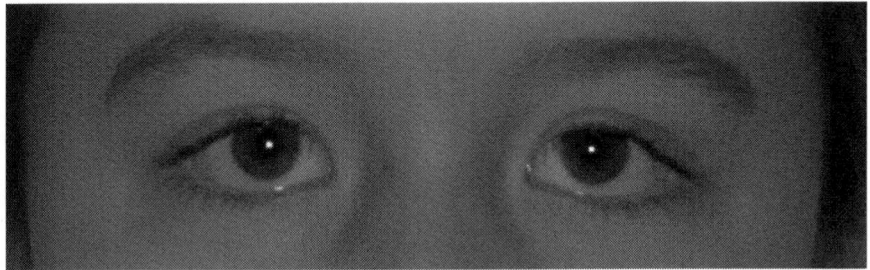

Mallampati Score. This grading system helps classify the degree of crowding in the oral airway. The more crowded oral airways in Class III and IV are normally indicative of a deficiency of forward jaw development and can mean a child is more prone to obstructive sleep breathing.

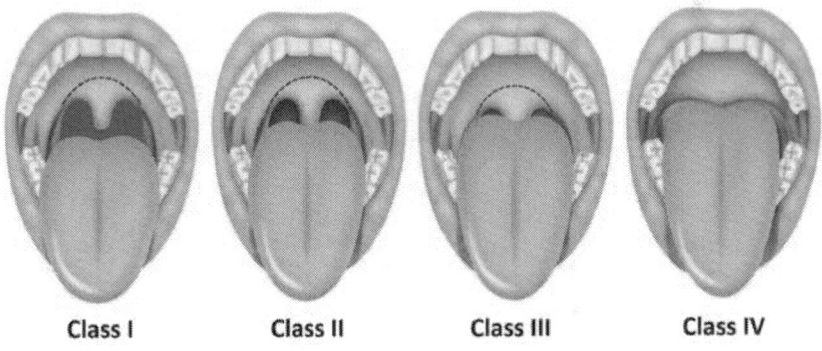

Class I   Class II   Class III   Class IV

Tonsil grading. This system helps classify the degree of enlargement of the tonsils. If a child has symptoms of abnormal breathing and tonsillar enlargement of Grade 3 or 4, an ENT referral may be warranted. Just as important as the size of the tonsils is how well the reflexes are working to keep the airway open during sleep – so it is not a completely linear relationship or indicator of problems.

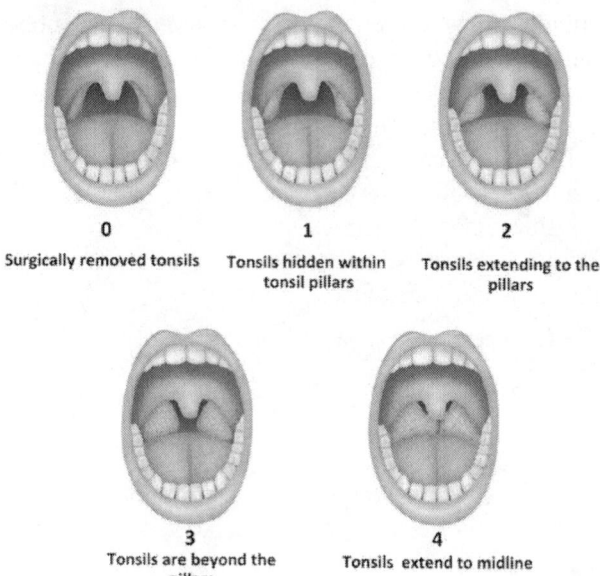

0	1	2
Surgically removed tonsils	Tonsils hidden within tonsil pillars	Tonsils extending to the pillars

3	4
Tonsils are beyond the pillars	Tonsils extend to midline

Narrow high palate. A high and narrow palate is linked to narrow nasal passages and reduced tongue space and is a well-established risk factor for sleep disturbed breathing from infancy to adulthood.

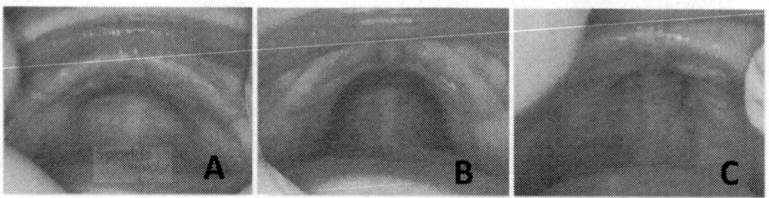

Normal (A) to high palates (B and C)

The palate is molded by the tongue early on in life, and if the palate is deep, narrowed, or V-shaped in contrast to U-shaped, it reflects an underlying dysfunction of the tongue. This is another risk factor for breathing difficulties.

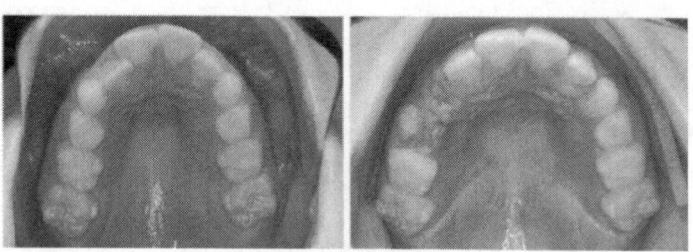

Narrow V-shaped palate (left) converted to a more normal U-shaped palate (right) with orthodontic treatment.

Orthodontic problems. As we discussed in the last chapter, orthodontic problems including crooked teeth most often reflect poor jaw development. This means reduced nasal passages, reduced tongue space, and reduced structural support of the throat muscles, all of which are known risk factors for sleep disturbed breathing across all ages.

Here is a summary of some of the common bite problems (from last chapter) that can be detectable long before the adult teeth come through. Children should have spaces between their baby teeth for their adult teeth to come through. If they don't, that is a sign of compromised airflow.

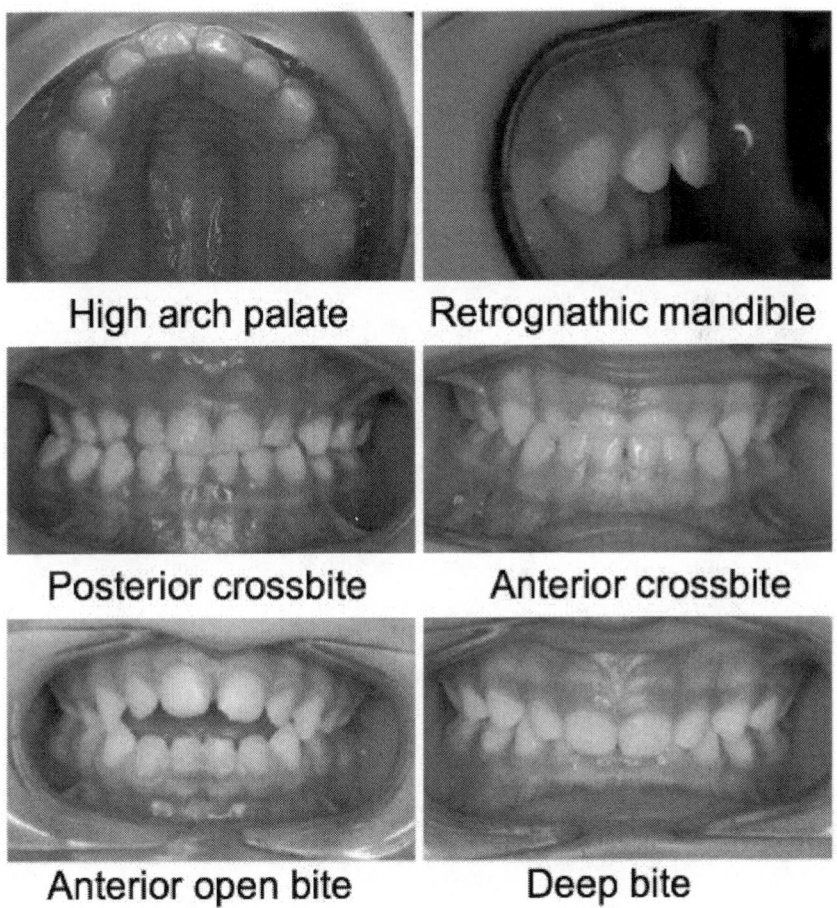

High arch palate   Retrognathic mandible

Posterior crossbite   Anterior crossbite

Anterior open bite   Deep bite

Tongue assessment. How the tongue sits in the mouth is another important element. Does it sit low between the teeth, or are the edges scalloped? Is there a tongue-tie?

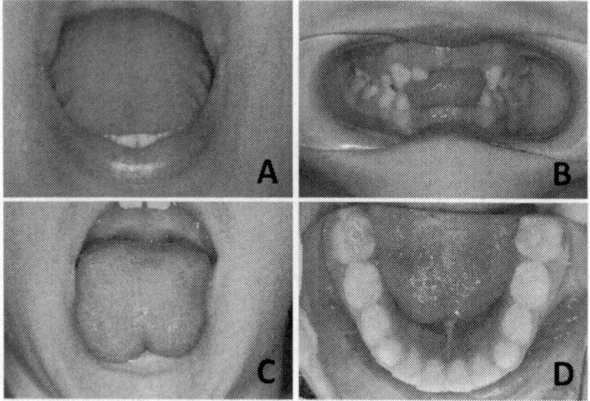

- Image A shows a scalloped tongue – tooth indents on the sides of the tongue indicate lowered tongue posture. Research has linked this with increased risk of disturbed breathing during sleep.[12]
- Image B shows a tongue thrust swallow – the tongue protrudes forward against the teeth during a swallow – this reflects lowered resting posture of the tongue.
- Images C and D show obvious or anterior tongue-ties – the image on the left depicts a classic heart-shaped indent on the tip of the tongue when it protrudes. The right image depicts a classic anterior tongue-tie where the tip of the tongue is attached to the floor of the mouth.

Tooth wear related to teeth grinding. Teeth grinding in children is a strong red flag for breathing difficulties during sleep.[13] In many cases, it is thought to be a compensation for airway narrowing and airflow restriction during sleep.[14-15] These occlusions are associated with brief arousals from sleep lasting a few seconds where the brain, heart, and breathing are reactivated and there is a rise in the muscle tone of the jaw muscles.[16] This muscle activity is thought to offer some protection against the severe collapses of the airway that define obstructive sleep apnoea. However, it is still linked to chronic activation of our "fight or flight" or stress response and unrestorative sleep.

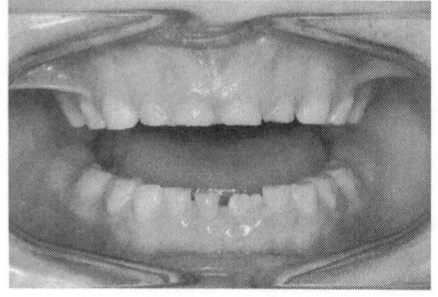

Recent research from UCLA associated sleep bruxism (teeth grinding) with low tongue posture, which can be attributed to nasal obstruction, enlarged tonsils, or restricted tongue mobility.[17] Research has also found that up to two-thirds of children who have their adenoids and tonsils surgically removed will have resolution of their teeth grinding after surgery.[18-19] I do often see children with persistent grinding after this surgery but have found that addressing constricted palates and tongue ties can be a missing link that may help resolve this issue.

Other known risk factors for teeth grinding include anti-depressants and stimulant medications. In these cases, it is still worthwhile to rule out breathing disturbances during sleep as these are linked to depression and ADHD symptoms in children.

If there are no linked breathing disturbances, in some cases no other intervention will be required, and a watchful waiting approach can be adopted.

Dental wear related to acid erosion. In children, acid wear would most commonly be related to airway or laryngopharyngeal reflux. Increased resistance to airflow results in increased effort to breathe and this creates negative intrathoracic pressures. This sucks up stomach juices, which aerosolise the acid and enzymes into the lungs and airway. This type of reflux can be associated with hoarseness, throat clearing and constant cough. These symptoms may sometimes lead to a misdiagnosis of asthma.

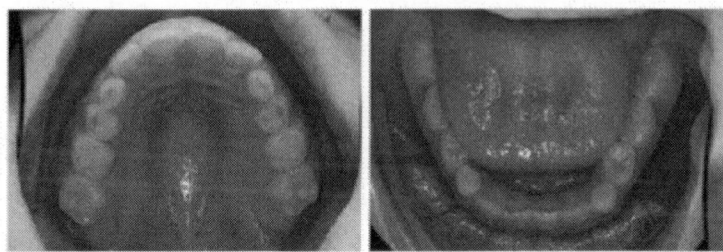

The aerosolised acid can go up into the sinuses and present as sinus headaches. It can also end up in the mouth, where its pH of 5.5 will be very damaging to dental health. Aerosolisation of acid is associated with increased risk of dental decay and gum inflammation, and acceleration of sleep bruxism-related tooth wear.[20]

Dental disease. Children who breathe through their mouths during sleep may be more prone to dental diseases such as gingivitis or inflammation of the gums and dental decay. This is because the mouth becomes dry, and the protective properties of saliva are lost. Saliva helps to cleanse the teeth and bacterial plaque, and it buffers the acids that break down the tooth structure.

It also has antimicrobial properties, plus contains important minerals required to remineralise the teeth following initial decay. Some children who have reflux disease as described above will have a highly acidic environment in the mouth, which favours the bacteria responsible for dental decay. A dry mouth also favours more of the bacteria that are likely to create inflammation in the gums.

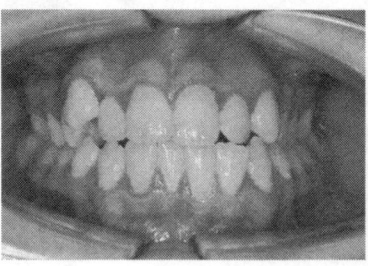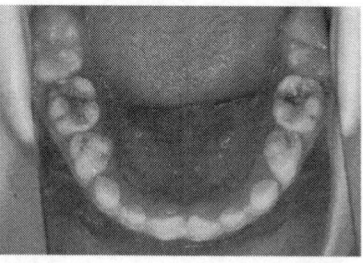

Missing teeth. Teeth missing from birth or removed to relieve dental crowding have been associated with mouth breathing and sleep disturbed breathing as well. This is because the growth of the jawbone is dependent on the presence of teeth. If they are not there, the jaws will be underdeveloped, and the dental arch will be more prone to collapsing. Dr Guilleminualt and team demonstrated this in a study of 31 children with congenitally missing teeth and 11 children who had permanent teeth extracted, and found all experienced a smaller overall oral cavity, leading to the collapse of the upper airway during sleep and OSA.[21]

Based on a combination of signs and symptoms of poor sleep and intra-oral findings, a dentist with an interest in airways will determine your child's risk of airway problems. If there are concerns, your child may be referred for a sleep study, ENT consultation, orthodontic treatment, or myofunctional therapy.

It's extremely important to have screenings done for your child if they present any of the warning signs of airway heath issues. The problems can compound quickly, and treatment is simpler with less irreversible consequences if it is timely.

SLEEP STUDIES FOR CHILDREN

A sleep study, or polysomnogram, helps to give more details about a child's sleep. It is often performed in a hospital setting overnight.

Sleep studies may not always be practical or easily available for children, and for this reason: The Pediatric Sleep Questionnaire (PSQ), shown below, is a 22-question scale, and positive answers to seven or more of these questions may be predictive of a diagnosis of sleep disturbed breathing based on a sleep study.[22] At the same time, it is not sensitive enough to predict milder breathing disturbances or mouth breathing, and so some children will remain undertreated if we rely on this alone.

Pediatric Sleep Questionnaire: Sleep-Disordered Breathing Subscale

070129

Child's Name: _____   Study ID #: _____

Person completing form: _____   Date: ___/___/___

Please answer these questions regarding the behavior of your child during sleep and wakefulness. The questions apply to how your child acts in general during the past month, not necessarily during the past few days since these may not have been typical if your child has not been well. You should circle the correct response or *print* your answers neatly in the space provided. A "Y" means "yes," "N" means "no," and "DK" means "don't know."

1. WHILE SLEEPING, DOES YOUR CHILD:
   - Snore more than half the time?...........................Y   N   DK | A2
   - Always snore? ....Y   N   DK | A3
   - Snore loudly? ....Y   N   DK | A4
   - Have "heavy" or loud breathing? ....Y   N   DK | A5
   - Have trouble breathing, or struggle to breathe? .....Y   N   DK | A6

2. HAVE YOU EVER SEEN YOUR CHILD STOP BREATHING DURING THE NIGHT? ....Y   N   DK | A7

3. DOES YOUR CHILD:
   - Tend to breathe through the mouth during the day?....Y   N   DK | A24
   - Have a dry mouth on waking up in the morning? ......Y   N   DK | A25
   - Occasionally wet the bed? ....Y   N   DK | A32

4. DOES YOUR CHILD:
   - Wake up feeling unrefreshed in the morning? ....Y   N   DK | B1
   - Have a problem with sleepiness during the day? ......Y   N   DK | B2

5. HAS A TEACHER OR OTHER SUPERVISOR COMMENTED THAT YOUR CHILD APPEARS SLEEPY DURING THE DAY? ....Y   N   DK | B4

6. IS IT HARD TO WAKE YOUR CHILD UP IN THE MORNING? ....Y   N   DK | B6

7. DOES YOUR CHILD WAKE UP WITH HEADACHES IN THE MORNING?.....Y   N   DK | B7

8. DID YOUR CHILD STOP GROWING AT A NORMAL RATE AT ANY TIME SINCE BIRTH? ....Y   N   DK | B9

9. IS YOUR CHILD OVERWEIGHT? ....Y   N   DK | B22

10. THIS CHILD **OFTEN**:
    - Does not seem to listen when spoken to directly. ......Y   N   DK | C3
    - Has difficulty organizing tasks and activities. ....Y   N   DK | C5
    - Is easily distracted by extraneous stimuli. ....Y   N   DK | C8
    - Fidgets with hands or feet or squirms in seat. ....Y   N   DK | C10
    - Is "on the go" or often acts as if "driven by a motor". ...Y   N   DK | C14
    - Interrupts or intrudes on others (eg., butts into conversations or games). ....Y   N   DK | C18

Thank you!

Be aware of the limitations of sleep study results.

Despite the vast quantity of information about a child's breathing and sleep every minute of the night, one of the limitations to be aware of relating to sleep study interpretation is that a child's diagnosis is often based on a single final number –the Apnoea Hypopnea Index (AHI). This is a summary of the total number of apnoeas or hypopneas per hour of sleep. That is, there is a focus on looking for the blockages of the airway that last ten seconds or more. Airway blockages must last ten seconds or more to be included in the score, even though shorter obstructive events can still be linked to increased work of breathing, fragmented and unrestorative sleep, and poor daytime function. A narrow focus on the AHI means that a lot of children with significant breathing disturbances and symptoms remain untreated and at risk of detrimental consequences.

Whilst an adult requires a very arbitrary five or more of these events per hour for a diagnosis, a child only requires one per hour based on their sensitivity to oxygen deprivation. It's not uncommon for me to receive a report concluding no OSA and no treatment required in a child even with an AHI of for example 1.6/hr.

In addition, for a hypopnea or partial blockage of the airway to be included, there must be a 4% drop in blood oxygenation and/or an arousal from sleep. This criterion was initially developed for the diagnosis of adults, but children do not tend to have as severe drops of oxygenation when their airway is blocked.

OSA pioneer Dr Christian Guilleminault and his team at Stanford Medical Centre developed a more sensitive "Stanford criteria" to help avoid underscoring of breathing problems. They counted ten second partial collapses of the airway with a 3% (not 4%) drop in oxygenation.

The team published a retrospective study where they followed up with 99 children who had a diagnosis of OSA using their sensitive criteria and had enlarged adenoids and tonsils removed to address this.[23] They then reviewed the original sleep study data and re-scored the AHI using the Academy of Sleep Medicine (AASM) criteria that is used more widely – including in sleep labs in Australia. They found that only nine of those 99 children would have been scored with a diagnosis of OSA.

Following surgery, all 99 children had improvement of their symptoms, ranging from snoring, pauses in breathing, gasping, excessive drooling, sweating, restlessness, teeth grinding, difficulties falling back to sleep, headaches, daytime fatigue, and sleepiness.

In addition, 22 out of 24 children who had been medicated with stimulants for ADHD symptoms had improvements in symptoms to the degree they could cease medications. All 33 of the children taking medications or sleeping aids were able to discontinue use.

Dr Guilleminault often spoke of his regret for establishing the AHI to define the severity of OSA and the focus it created on very arbitrary cut-offs. By the end of his career, based on the research described above, he was advocating for more attention to the restrictions in airflow even in the absence of oxygen deprivation.

> The take-home lesson for parents if your child is having a sleep study is to understand that AHI is a very insensitive marker of breathing problems, and that any snoring should still be investigated and addressed.

It is not uncommon practice for an ENT surgeon to go straight to removing obstructive adenoids and tonsils without a sleep study if a child has no significant medical conditions or syndromes and there is snoring and other symptoms of disturbed breathing during sleep present.

Along the same lines, I do not necessarily require a sleep study to justify addressing the risk factor of narrow palate/narrow nasal floor with palate expansion.

Before I launch into more details about referral pathways to address the various risk factors in the next few chapters, I want to briefly mention a commonly prescribed treatment option for obstructive breathing in children.

CONTINUOUS POSITIVE AIRWAY PRESSURE

Continuous positive airway pressure (CPAP) uses a machine that delivers a constant and steady air pressure via a hose and facemask to splint the airway open and prevent collapse.

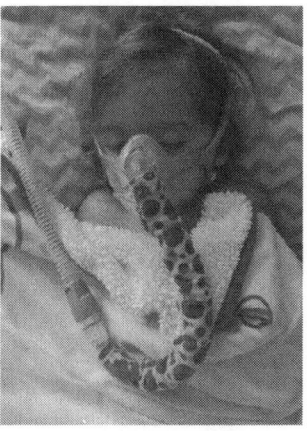

Parent photo used with consent

An overlooked problem with using CPAP in children is the impact on the growing face. In orthodontics, it is understood that bone movement is influenced by the duration, frequency, and intensity of force application. Since CPAP is utilized all night long, on a nightly basis, and with a firm fit to avoid leakage of air, there is a strong potential to influence growth of the facial bone structures. CPAP forces retard forward development of the midface– a key area that needs to be developed in these children to help create space for the airway.[24]

> **Despite the improvements in quality of life, CPAP is nothing more than a band-aid solution to address symptoms and lacks precision in targeting specific risk factors.**

It may have a role in helping children with genetic, craniofacial, or neuromuscular syndromes, but it is best reserved as a crutch until a better airway can be developed through growth modification with orthodontic appliances.

• • •

I've mentioned several practices throughout the chapters in Part I that promote good airway health from birth. These include breastfeeding, baby-led weaning, chewing hard foods, and avoiding pacifiers, sippy cups, and pouch foods when children are babies.

However, as children grow and showcase signs related to compromised airway health, some of the practices to help get your child back on track include removal of their adenoids and tonsils, palate expansion, myofunctional therapy, and tongue tie release. Often, it will take an integrative team approach to screen, address, and correct any functional or structural disorders that are contributing. In the following chapters, I will expand on these in more detail so you can contribute to the discussion of what may be best for your child.

8

ADENOIDS, TONSILS, AND GROMMETS

One of the key people on your child's airway health team will be an Ear, Nose and Throat (ENT) surgeon. This chapter will give you an overview of some of their most performed procedures, including removal of adenoid and tonsils, turbinate reduction, and placement of ear tubes or grommets. It's important to understand that the ultimate outcome for all children is to restore nasal breathing and that treatment does not start and end with an ENT surgeon. Even after surgery, many children will still require a team approach to restoring proper airway structure and nasal breathing.

The traditional thinking is that ENT problems like enlarged adenoids, tonsils and turbinates are root causes of breathing problems. However, recent research using objective data has confirmed surgery is not curative of breathing problems for most children. This chapter is about highlighting the new perspective that common ENT problems could be symptoms of a bigger problem: underlying airway dysfunction.

This means that instead of accepting the development of problems and the need for these common ENT surgeries as a rite of passage, we can better identify red flags of future problems and set an alternative path to proactively reduce surgical needs for children in the future.

ADENOIDS AND TONSILS

Adenoids and tonsils are masses of lymphoid tissue that are found on the sides of the neck inside the throat. They are the body's first line of defence against foreign materials (like allergens, cigarette smoke, and environmental pollution) and pathogens that enter through the nose and mouth. They capture and trap these materials when they enter the airway and activate an immune response that helps fight bacteria and viruses before they can spread into the body.

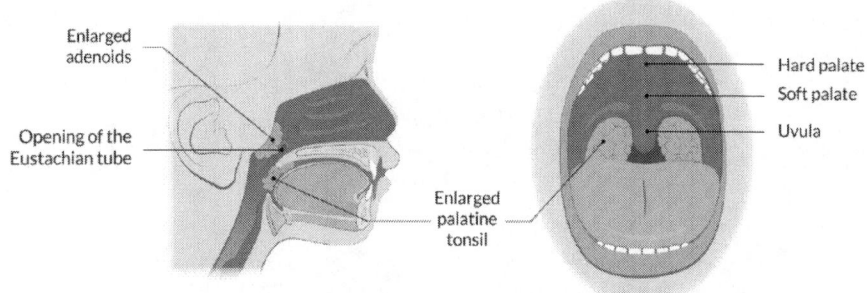

The adenoids sit higher at the back of the nose. They can be visualised with a nasoendoscope – a thin, flexible tube with a camera and light at the end that is inserted through the nose and into the throat. They can also be viewed on some x-ray images. The palatine tonsils can often be visualized just by looking inside the mouth to the back of the throat.

If these tissues overgrow, they may become more problematic than beneficial.

There are two main problems with the adenoids and tonsils that can significantly decrease a child's quality of life.

The first is recurrent throat infections. Guidelines from the American Academy of Otolaryngology-Head and Neck Surgery strongly recommend "watchful waiting" rather than opting for surgery to remove the tonsils and adenoids if there have been seven or less episodes in the past year, five or less episodes in each of the past two years, or fewer than three episodes in the past three years.[1] This is a very high threshold for surgical intervention and may not be helpful for children who require multiple GP visits, courses of antibiotics, and days off school to recover (not to mention the days their parents must take off from work to take care of them).

But the second, bigger problem is that the **adenoids and tonsils can obstruct the airway and cause breathing difficulties, especially during sleep.** Some of the children with this issue will also have difficulties chewing and swallowing tough foods like meat.

That is why the same AAO-HNS guidelines suggest that if a child does not meet the criteria for removing them due to recurrent throat infections, caregivers need to also be asked about problems with snoring and obstructive breathing and associated conditions that may improve with removal, including growth retardation, poor school performance, bedwetting, asthma, and behavioural problems. If these issues are present, surgical removal could be considered despite the absence of throat infections.

The adenoid and tonsil tissues tend to peak in size around the age of two-six years – which is also the peak period for snoring and obstructive breathing during sleep. Sometimes the professional advice is that children will grow out of it. But the reality is that if young children are chronically snoring, they may be growing *into* it.

This is because children have the highest need for restorative sleep in the early years of life. The brain is going through a critical period of development, and compelling research suggests that snoring children are at greater risk of grey matter loss, as well as neurocognitive, socio-emotional, and behavioural problems. This risk can be persistent even after the snoring subsides. We have no way of knowing which individual children will be affected most.

In the past, the main reason for the removal of tonsils was to prevent recurrent throat infections. Research by Erikson et al. identified an increasing rate of removal of these tissues between 1970 and 2005.[2] In 1970, 88.4% of these surgeries were done for infection-related reasons. In 2005, the majority (76.8%) were instead primarily performed to help resolve obstructive breathing.

If your child has enlarged tonsils and you become concerned about their breathing during sleep, one of the things that can happen if you go to a GP for an ENT referral is that they will say there have not been enough episodes of recurrent tonsillitis to warrant this. You will need to find an airway-aware medical or dental professional to help with the referral.

Traditional options can include surgical removal of obstructive adenoids and tonsils, or a short-term trial of anti-inflammatory medications to see if swelling can be reduced. Although surgery does come with risks, in some cases these are outweighed by the potential benefits. These procedures have been linked to improvements in:

- behavioural and neurocognitive problems – both subjective and by test scores
- school performance
- bedwetting
- height, weight, and growth
- asthma outcomes – less medication, emergency room visits for asthma related symptoms, overall asthma symptoms, and asthma exacerbations

However, current thinking is that, despite the immediate improvement in symptoms, removing tonsils and adenoids is not the magic cure that it was once thought to be.

One of the most significant studies that looked at before and after objective sleep study results in 578 children across eight sleep centres in the U.S. and Europe found that, while the children's breathing had generally improved, only 27% had complete resolution of obstructive sleep apnoea.[3]

There was an average reduction of OSA or AHI from 18.2 to 4.1. This means despite symptomatic improvements, an average child still had four blockages to air flow lasting ten seconds or more per hour of sleep. The main factors associated with persistent problems were:

- obesity
- older age (being over seven years)
- asthma
- allergic rhinitis
- bedwetting
- increased severity of OSA before surgery

The risk of persistent problems in older childhood is thought to be related to the alterations in normal jaw development that have occurred with mouth breathing and low tongue posture by the time they reach that age.

Furthermore, other studies are showing that, in children who have initial resolution, symptoms and obstructive sleep apnoea may return later in childhood.

One of the main problems that I manage in my practice is persistent mouth breathing or snoring in children after surgery. These children may present with parents who have ongoing concerns about their child's sleep, behaviour, concentration, and attention. Some of these children have even had repeat operations because the tissues regrew.

A key message for parents is that removal of obstructive adenoids and tonsils can play a very important role in improving your child's breathing, as it effectively unclogs the airway. It can offer immediate benefits in terms of quality of life but is not a blanket solution.

Taking out enlarged adenoids and tonsils is like taking furniture out of a small room. It will make it less crowded and easier for air to flow through, but it can be equally important to remodel or expand the room. This can be done through guiding facial development forward and wide with orthodontic intervention, including palate expansion. It is also important to address any allergies or other sources of inflammation and swelling and restore normal nasal breathing and tongue and throat muscle function through myofunctional therapy (Chapter 11). This may include releasing tongue ties that restrict normal mobility of the tongue and hinder a child's capacity to restore normal muscle patterns.

Getting to the root of swollen adenoids and tonsils

Earlier, in Chapter 6, I discussed how crooked teeth have become so prevalent that braces are considered a rite of passage for most children. The conventional approach to orthodontics treats the symptom rather than any underlying cause. There is a reliance on retainer wear to maintain results; even so, it's not uncommon for results to relapse and teeth to become crooked again.

The situation with removing adenoids and tonsils has some parallels. Each year in the US, 300,000 children under 15 years have their adenoids and tonsils removed. This number is closer to 48,000 in Australia.

It's a procedure not without risks, including bleeding and use of general anaesthetic. And yet, a large part of my work is managing children who have persistent breathing problems after surgery or need to have the operation redone when they are older.

This is the reason that we must get to the root of the problem and identify what contributes to some children having obstruction to see if we can potentially avoid it.

The conventional view is that overgrowth of adenoids and tonsils is due to some sort of inflammatory response from viruses, cigarette smoke, allergies, or aerosolised acids with reflux disease. Anti-inflammatory medications are sometimes offered, which may or may not help with the situation.

Under this model, the enlargement causes airway narrowing and mouth breathing, which alters the way the jaw and facial structures grow, resulting in an "adenoids facies" facial pattern. This is characterized by narrow palates, longer faces, and receded lower jaws. These changes are subtle or subclinical, so they may not always be recognizable.

This assumption is that sleep disturbed breathing is caused by the narrow airway – from both the swollen soft tissue inside and underdevelopment of the jaws which form the outer framework.

However, over a lifetime of research, the late Stanford sleep medicine and obstructive sleep apnoea pioneer Dr Christian Guilleminault proposed an alternative view– that the subtle underdevelopment of the bony structures that support the nose and throat contributes to mouth breathing and that the enlarged adenoids and tonsils are just symptoms along the way.

This line of thinking has been further validated by the work of ENT/Facial Plastic Surgeon Dr Howard Stupak.[4,5] His published work supports that the problem starts with poor nasal airflow. The increased effort of breathing through the narrowed nasal airway creates a vacuum pressure (much the same as sucking too hard on a straw would cause it to collapse), and this repetitive pressure damages the throat wall and leads to inflammation and stretching of the adenoids and tonsils inside the airway. This leads to continued mouth breathing, which perpetuates the cycle of poor jaw development.

Because I see so many children with persistent or recurrent problems even after removal of adenoids and tonsils, and because I have witnessed the positive impact that orthodontic treatment has on these symptoms, I tend to support this alternative hypothesis.

> **We need to pay attention to the more subtle underdeveloped palates and limitations in nasal airflow that occur long before obstructive sleep apnoea develops.**

The pioneering researchers on palate expansion for children with obstructive sleep apnoea observed that enlarged adenoids and tonsils shrunk during orthodontic treatment. More recent work published in early 2022 by orthodontists Drs. Audrey Yoon and Rebecca Bockow found that children aged 7-8 years with enlarged adenoids and tonsils and high palates who underwent palate expansion had significant reduction in the volume of their adenoids and tonsils compared to children who had no treatment.[6] These children also had improvement in their symptoms of disrupted breathing during sleep, which could be related to their improved airflow.

If the tonsils are not excessively large, palate expansion may be a reasonable first step before jumping straight into surgery.

In my practice, I often offer expansion and ENT referral at the same time if the tonsils are Grade 3 or less and a child can breathe reasonably with their mouth closed. I know there will usually be some breathing improvement within six weeks of commencing palate expansion, and there may be a longer wait to get to see an ENT or even schedule surgery, so providing both options simultaneously offer children and parents a chance to see how much the child's breathing and daytime issues can be resolved with expansion and whether surgery can be avoided.

Even when we can improve airway structure with surgical removal of enlarged adenoids and tonsils and palate expansion, Dr Guilleminault's work suggests the only valid finish line is ensuring nasal breathing.[7] We need to re-educate children to close their mouths, keep their tongues up, and breathe through their noses for better airflow.

TURBINATES

While we're on the topic of ENT surgery, I'm going to discuss turbinate reduction, which is another commonly offered surgery to improve nasal airflow.

The turbinates are projections of bones in the nasal cavity which help slow down the passage of air before it enters the body so it can be better warmed, humidified, and filtered.

They can become swollen and enlarged, and removal may be recommended at the time of removing the adenoids and tonsils. Often, the enlargement is thought to be a symptom of allergies, and the assumption is that these are the origin of poor nasal airflow, despite studies showing no direct correlation between allergies and the size of the turbinates.

Once again, Dr Stupak questions conventional thinking and hypothesizes enlarged turbinates could be a compensation for nasal disuse.[5] That is, when individuals don't use their nose to breathe, there is a negative or suction pressure created in the nose when air flows down the throat. This causes stretching and pulling of the turbinate tissues into the nasal cavity where there is low airflow.

One of the side effects of reducing the turbinates is variations of what is called "Empty Nose Syndrome." Over-reduction of the turbinates can lead to varying degrees of stagnated airflow. Dr Stupak provides the analogy of canoeing down a flowing river and encountering a lake opening. Rather than being able to flow smoothly down the river, there will be a circular current and stagnation. When airflow isn't directed smoothly, symptoms include nasal dryness and crusting and a sensation of being unable to breathe well.

Nasal breathing has been shown to reduce symptoms of allergic rhinitis. Research from Perth from the 1970's demonstrated that children who had palate expansion due to allergic rhinitis (in other words, for reasons that were totally not about the teeth) could breathe more effectively through their nose and had reduction in allergic symptoms.[8]

We need to keep questioning root causes and promoting nasal breathing as early as possible to minimize problems.

MIDDLE EAR INFECTIONS AND GLUE EAR

Lastly, to finish off this chapter, I want to spend some time talking about middle ear infections and glue ear.

Ear infections are the most common problem that children present to their medical practitioner with. They are common reasons for antibiotic use, which can have a huge impact on children's gut bacteria and health. As a dentist, I'm also concerned with the risks of disturbance to the enamel formation as their teeth develop. Again, we need to look at root causes here.

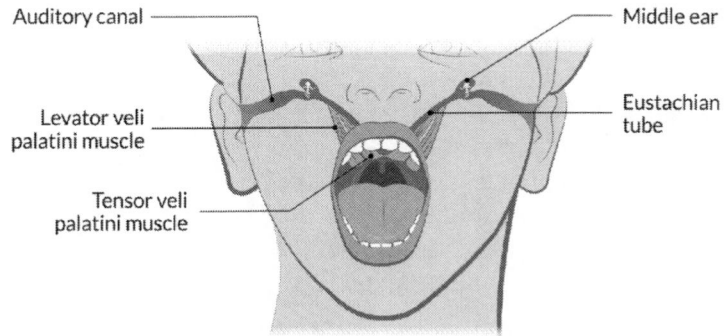

Young children are most prone to ear infections because their eustachian tubes, which clear secretions from the middle ear to the back of the nose, are more underdeveloped and horizontal. When these tubes don't work properly, they may become more contaminated with bacteria and viruses at the back of the nose where the adenoids sit. Enlarged adenoids create the perfect storm for acute middle ear infections.

Other times, there is chronic build-up of non-infected fluid in the ear which can lead to conductive hearing loss. Grommets, or tiny plastic ear tubes, are placed surgically in the eardrum to help the fluid drain. Infection can also drain out through the grommet. This can help children hear again, which is incredibly important for their speech development.

However, grommets can fall out, and what I see are children who have had repeated tubes placed. I know at least two children who have had six sets of grommets placed. One of them had a perforated eardrum from one of her surgeries and now must wear a hearing aid. The risk of damage or scarring on this delicate part of the ear with repeated surgeries and the long-term impact on hearing concerns me.

Like the adenoids and tonsils, turbinate surgeries have a role in significantly improving quality of life. But let's look beyond the surgery and address underlying root causes.

I see a lot of infants in my practice for tongue tie release, and I can usually predict which children are going to be prone to ear infections. Research tells us that children with a high, narrow palate are three and a half times more likely to have an ear infection during their first year of life.[9] These children will also be two and a half times more likely to require grommets or ear tubes by the age of four years.

This is because good swallowing is essential for the eustachian tube to work and drain properly. Many of us can relate to this when we're on a plane and we need a good swallow to equalise pressure in our ears.

A narrow, high palate means reduced structural support for the soft palate. The muscles that elevate the soft palate are also involved in dilating or opening the eustachian tube. So, a narrow palate could alter swallowing and contribute to poor eustachian tube function.

We also know pacifier use, which alters swallowing patterns, is linked to increased risk of ear infections.

Several studies have shown that palate expansion can improve conductive hearing loss in children with glue ear.[10-11] There is even one study by Kılıç and team that randomized children into two groups – one group had grommets, the other had palate expansion.[11] Both groups had hearing improvements in the same range. Based on these findings, the researchers suggested that palate expansion would be the preferable option.

They also published further research in 2021 that demonstrated improvements in eustachian tube function using objective measures with palate expansion.[12]

> These common ENT surgeries is that that they can be helpful to buy time until a child is ready to address the underlying problem more definitively, but we do need to look at the bigger picture and address root causes – especially if your child needs to have any surgery more than once.

In the future, there will be greater attention to good jaw development and airway function, and this may help minimize the need for surgery in the first place.

Palate expansion has a very important role in combination with ENT surgeries to improve nasal airflow, and it can also help with optimizing the bony structures for better swallowing and eustachian tube function. The next chapter will cover what all parents need to know about palate expansion.

9

PALATE EXPANSION

Traditionally, palate expansion has been reserved to help address orthodontic problems like dental crowding and crossbites in growing children. These days, there is mounting evidence that this orthodontic intervention can play a central role in restoring nasal breathing and tongue space – and may even help alleviate snoring or obstructive sleep apnoea in both children and adults.

In this chapter, we will explore how palate expansion works, what the different available options are, and how you can use this information to best support your child's needs.

As dentists, we are taught that the best time to begin palate expansion for children is around the age of seven to eight years, and that we should refer a child for their first orthodontic evaluation by the age of seven years.

What I was finding was that once the child had been seen by an orthodontist, they were most often scheduled for regular observation until the age of around 12 years, when their teeth would be straightened with braces. Around that time we would often receive requests to extract premolar teeth to alleviate dental crowding before the braces were put on, so the teeth could be straightened with maximum efficiency.

Around ten years ago, when I first learned that palate expansion could help children breathe better and have functional benefits far beyond straight teeth, I decided I was going to dive deeper. I remember the sense of anxiety that came from extracting healthy permanent teeth. Pulling them was traumatizing not only for the child, but for me, as well. I knew I didn't want this for my own kids, which made guiding good jaw growth even more compelling.

When I see my adult OSA patients, I am so disheartened to hear of all the challenges they experience and see their narrow palates, which are more complex to modify in adulthood.

To this day, there is still conflicting information about this option. My aim is to present why it's important, so that you as a parent can weigh up all perspectives to make a fully informed decision.

WHAT IS THE SIGNIFICANCE OF A NARROW PALATE?

Narrow palates have been well established as a risk factor for sleep disturbed breathing in infancy through to adulthood. As we have discussed, the palate, or roof of the mouth, is the floor of the nose and sinus areas. If this area is narrow, it causes a dramatic reduction in the cross section of the nasal airway. This is represented by the boxes in the following image.

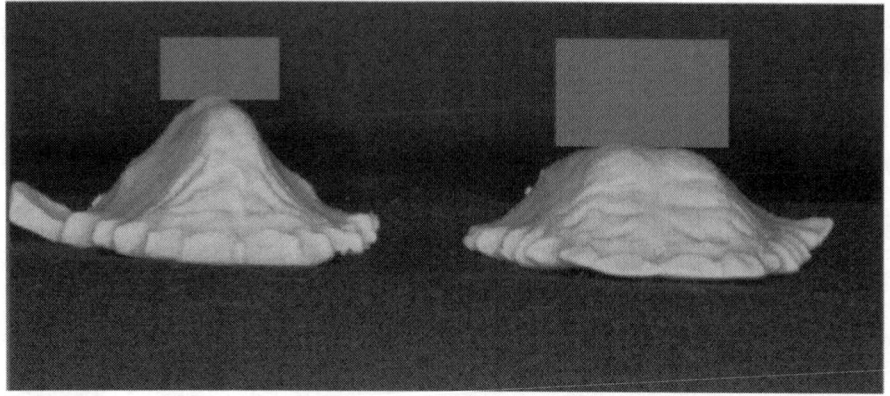

Image shared and used with permission by Dr Karen O'Rourke

Increased resistance to nasal airflow predisposes a person to mouth breathing and snoring, and increased collapsibility of the airway.

The problem of the narrow nasal airway can be compounded by a deviated nasal septum. The nasal septum forms the midline support of the nose, separating the right and left nostrils. It is composed of cartilage and bone towards the back. Deviated septums commonly occur in association with high, narrow palates. The septum is fixed in size, and buckles as it has to fit into a more compact space. This can further narrow the airway and increase resistance to breathing on the side it deviates into.

Narrow palates also reduce space for normal tongue to palate contact, which is associated with stable breathing during sleep. In growing children, this tongue to palate contact at rest is critical for stimulating proper palate development. In general, narrow palates perpetuate a cycle of oral dysfunction, and poor structural development.

PALATE EXPANSION FOR BETTER BREATHING

Palate expansion has been established as an option to help improve nasal breathing for over 100 years. Even relatively minor amounts of palate expansion (in the range of a few millimetres) have been demonstrated to increase the cross section of the nasal airway and exponentially improve nasal airflow.

One of the most significant studies on the impact of palate expansion on nasal breathing was conducted in Perth at our local children's hospital, Princess Margaret Hospital, by ENT surgeon Dr Lindsay Gray.[1] This study, published in 1975 in an international ENT journal, included 310 consecutive children who were treated with palate expansion for medical reasons in a collaboration between Gray and orthodontist Dr Bill Brogan. The medical reasons for intervention included:

- poor nasal airway
- nasal septal deformity
- recurrent ear, nasal, or sinus infections
- allergic rhinitis
- asthma
- prior to septoplasty (surgical correction of a deviated nasal septum)

Dr Gray found that 87% of these children changed from mouth to nasal breathing and ceased to be noisy sleepers. The ones that didn't make the change had more severe nasal septum deformations or severe allergies. There was also an improvement in colds and respiratory infections, nasal allergies, and many cases of asthma across the board. He concluded that palate expansion was a comparatively simple and conservative method of treating impaired nasal breathing, even in the absence of an orthodontic problem

A more recent meta-analysis pooling data from 12 palate expansion studies measuring nasal airflow with rhinometry, confirmed reduced nasal resistance and improved nasal airflow with treatment.[2] We mustn't overlook the effectiveness of a palate expansion as a targeted intervention to improve nasal breathing

Based on evidence to support improved nasal breathing outcomes, researchers started investigating the role of palate expansion in reducing snoring and obstructive sleep apnoea at the turn of the century.

There is mounting data supporting its important role in helping to resolve sleep breathing difficulties[3,4] – especially in conjunction with surgical removal of enlarged adenoids and tonsils (which we went over in detail in the previous chapter).

When the palate is widened, more room is opened for the tongue to fit properly in the mouth. This allows for improvement in tongue posture, and the capacity to restore tongue to palate contact. As the tongue sits higher, the base of the tongue encroaches less on the upper airway.[5]

| In growing children, the improvements in tongue posture and tongue function can help stimulate more normal palate development.

This helps break the constant downward spiral of poor structure and function.

With increased tongue space, some parents also report their child spontaneously closes their mouth more or speaks more clearly, within one to two months, even whilst the orthodontic device is still in their mouth. In addition, muscles of the upper airway that attach to the palate have increased support and tension. This reduces collapsibility of the throat part of the upper airway during sleep.

There are other secondary functional improvements commonly seen with palate expansion, such as the reduction of bed wetting and ear infections. The link with eustachian tubes was explored in the last chapter.

Bedwetting is a red flag for breathing disturbances during sleep. It has been commonly associated with nasal obstruction and obstructive sleep apnoea. There have been a few different mechanisms proposed, and it is likely to be a combination that contributes to bedwetting.

The sudden intrathoracic pressure changes that come from increased efforts to breathe cause pressure changes in the abdomen, affecting the bladder's capacity to hold urine. The increased stress and subsequent rise in systemic blood pressure leads to the release of a cascade of hormones that results in increased excretion of sodium and increased urine volumes.[6]

One study of 54 bedwetting children used sleep studies to determine that 68.5% of them had OSA.[7] Nasal obstruction and narrow high palate were common findings. Another contributing factor proposed for their bedwetting, was that these children have an increased arousal threshold and are deeper sleepers. This is in contrast to children with milder breathing disturbances who may be more responsive, arouse easily and work harder to breathe to keep their airway open.

Multiple studies have demonstrated that palate expansion can help eliminate bedwetting.[8,9] In practice, parents commonly report drier nappies or reduction or elimination of bedwetting within one to two months of treatment, including in children who have not responded well to the front-line option of electric alarms.

HOW IS THE PALATE WIDENED?

Palate expansion utilizes removable plates or fixed orthodontic appliances cemented in the mouth.

In children, the midline suture between the two halves of the palate is not completely fused, and it is possible to use these appliances supported on the teeth to apply a gentle force across the midline suture via a screw mechanism. This gently separates the halves of the palate, stimulating new bone formation in the region of the midline or nasal floor. This process is called "distraction osteogenesis."

There are many different expansion device designs, all of which work effectively in young children. Some practitioners are comfortable with fixed appliances like the banded hyrax and bonded hyrax which are cemented in the mouth and don't rely as much on good patient co-operation.

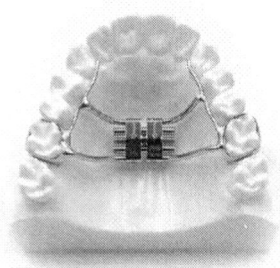 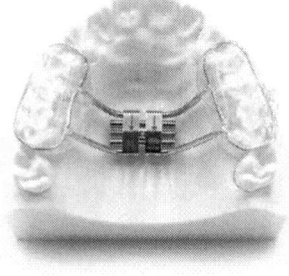

Banded Expander   Bonded Expander

Photos used with permission of Orthodent Laboratory

As a child reaches the age of around 10 to 12 years, when braces are normally considered, the midline suture becomes more fused, and the other bones of the face are more firmly set and the two halves of the palate resist separation. Expansion forces tend to tip the teeth outwards rather than stimulate new bone formation at the mid palate suture. This is called 'dental expansion' as opposed to 'bony expansion' or 'skeletal expansion.' This can create more space in the mouth, but it is highly unstable and does not produce the widened nasal floor necessary for optimal sleep and breathing outcomes.

If we miss the window of intervention in early childhood, it is still possible to achieve true bony expansion of the nasal floor using 'bone-borne expansion.' This means that, instead of using an appliance that is supported completely on the teeth, the expansion device is supported by mini-implants or temporary anchorage devices are placed in the bone close to the midline suture.

This allows the expansion force to be applied more directly across the suture as the screw mechanism is turned, reliably separating the mid-palate suture.

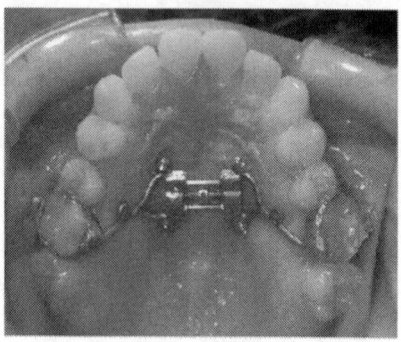

Photo used with permission by Dr Audrey Yoon

In young adults, the use of miniature implants can often eliminate the need for more invasive surgery in conjunction with palate expansion that is normally required to achieve similar outcomes for older adults. You can read more about new protocols that make it possible to achieve these outcomes for adults in Chapter 11.

In my practice I am focused on expansion for children ages nine and under. My personal preference is a removable expansion plate called the Biobloc Stage 1 Expander. This was developed by British orthodontist Dr John Mew who pioneered orthotropics – an approach to orthodontics which focuses on guiding facial growth forwards in conjunction with improving oral rest posture and tongue-to-palate contact.

In addition to the increased width, it also uses extra curved wires at the front of the mouth to control the entire arch form and alignment of the upper front teeth. With this device, we can usually achieve broader, well-aligned smiles at the same time as the expansion.

The appliances are well tolerated by most children, and they are worn all day, during eating and sleeping. The main advantage of removable devices is that they can be removed to clean and allow good dental hygiene.

Parents are instructed to turn the screw every night at the rate of 1/8 turn (1/8mm) per day. After the expansion is complete, the bony remodeling of the nasal floor tends to be stable, but the teeth positions are not. These are largely influenced by the balance between the muscles of lips, cheeks, and tongue.

Underlying poor oral posture and oral dysfunction do need to be addressed to ensure long-term stability of results. Once expansion is complete, we commence myofunctional therapy to restore normal lip seal, nasal breathing, tongue posture, and swallowing. Here's a case to illustrate the expander and typical result.

Case Study: Palate expansion for 8-year-old with sleep concerns

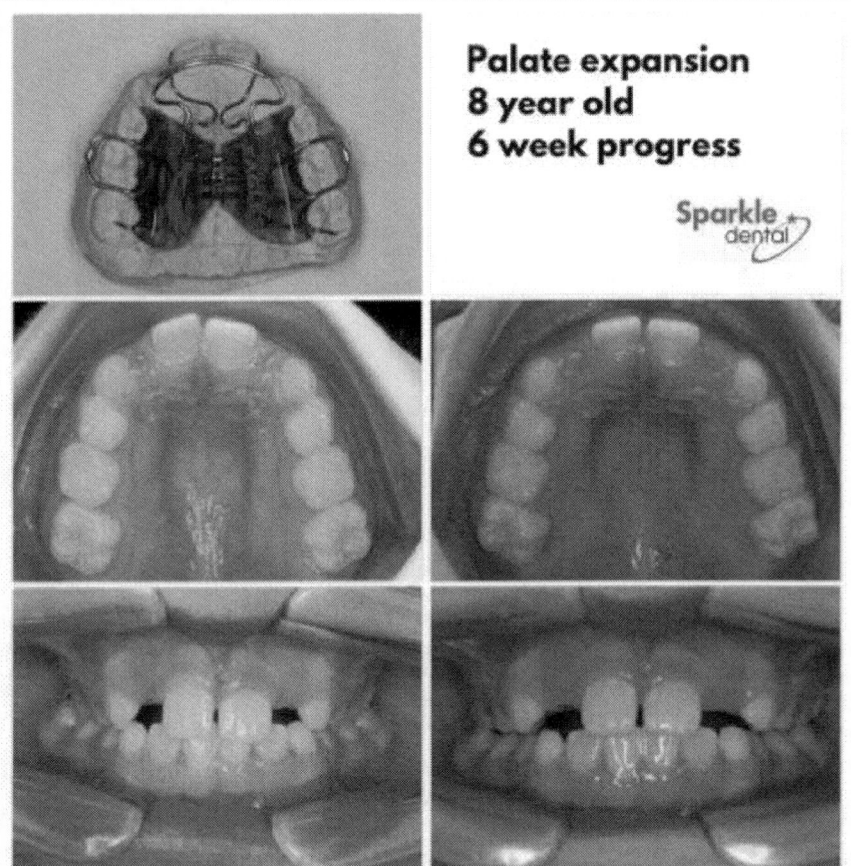

Palate expansion
8 year old
6 week progress

Sparkle
dental

The prompt for treatment for this patient was unrestorative sleep and concerns with daytime function. His treatment plan included palate expansion, followed by myofunctional therapy and adjunctive tongue-tie release.

At the six-week mark, there was significant remodeling of his nasal floor and an increase in tongue space evident.

His mum reported:
• Nasal breathing was easier – the mouth is closed more habitually.
• Patient is more refreshed on waking.
• No bedwetting since – was previously once per fortnight.
• More rested, especially after school – happy to play rather than wanting to chill.

122 | BREATHE, SLEEP, THRIVE

WHAT AGE CAN PALATE EXPANSION BE COMMENCED?

The traditional age to commence palate expansion is seven to eight years old, when the first permanent incisor teeth are starting to erupt. But I've started to question that tradition in recent years and have commenced palate expansion in children as young as three years of age.

It's become difficult to ignore the positive changes reported by parents – their child's speech seems clearer, they close their mouth more during sleep, teeth grinding and snoring is eliminated, they are sleeping more restfully, waking more refreshed, not as prone to tantrums and meltdowns, and have more energy to enjoy sports after school. Children become a bit easier to manage, and parents also enjoy seeing their broader smiles and fuller faces.

Ages seven to eight years is a very arbitrary barrier to commence treatment despite parents having significant functional concerns earlier. I decided to allow parents the choice to start early by offering palate expansion for those below the "traditional" age. One of the biggest obstacles when seeking care is finding professionals trained in orthodontics who are comfortable working with and managing such young children. I know this because it took our team practice and experience as we reduced our age threshold for patients. I know there will come a time I will feel more compelled and comfortable to commence treatment in even younger children. I see so many infants, I can identify the high arch palate from very early in life. I know these children are at greater risk of developing nasal disuse, snoring and obstructive breathing, and other functional issues like eustachian tube dysfunction, ear infections, and speech problems.

A child's greatest need for restorative sleep and peak window of brain development is before the age of three years.

If jaw development peaks before the age of six years, then we can best modify the narrow palate risk factor and optimize breathing, sleep, and oral function in the earliest years of life – well before the first six-year-old molar teeth come in.

Achieving optimal housing for the tongue ensures that we can interrupt the downward spiral of poor function and jaw development. Myofunctional therapy will be a critical piece of this puzzle to help restore this function after structural correction.

Case Study: palate expansion for 3.5-year-old with persistent sleep breathing disturbance following ENT surgery

Here are photos – pretreatment and at the 12-month review – of the very first three-year-old I offered palate expansion to in my practice.

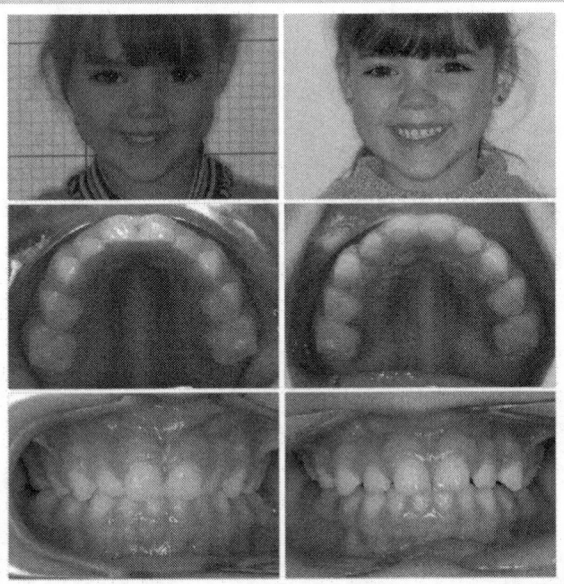

Her mum's initial concerns were persistent snoring, teeth grinding, and mouth breathing after two surgeries – one to remove her adenoids and insert grommets, and the other seven months later to remove her tonsils as they were told that would help her speech clarity. Her sleep was still very restless, and she was having nightmares at least twice a week. Mum could understand her speaking, but others had more trouble. Her regular dentist identified that the roof of her mouth was very narrow and referred her to our practice for assessment and expansion.

It's possible to see the spaces appearing between the front baby teeth, the remodeling that has occurred in the middle of the palate or nasal floor, and the increased tongue space and broader smile.

Sleep became less fragmented and more restorative. She is quieter, and she is not waking to come into mum's room in the middle of the night. Her grandmother commented that, before treatment, she had trouble understanding her. "When she started the treatment, we started to notice the improvement in speech – she never had any trouble talking. It was the way the words came out. A very intelligent girl whose words couldn't be heard, and now they can."

Surprisingly, around the time I began working with three-year-olds, I discovered an article published in 1922 in the Journal of the American Medical Association written by paediatrician Dr Samuel Cohen.[10]

He proposed his physician colleagues add a caliper to their tools and check the width of the palate in children. He also stated that the ideal time for orthodontic treatment was as early as possible, ideally around the age of 30 months and before the age of six years, whilst growth was still occurring rapidly, to optimize nasal breathing, eustachian tube function, hearing, and facial development. This window of 30 months is also significant because it corresponds to a rapid window of brain and general development

It's incredible to see how this has come full circle and I hope it doesn't take another one hundred years for this to catch on further.

Over the last couple of years, our team has become more comfortable working with younger children and with the idea of a longer journey of treatment and follow up. Thinking about the experiences that these children would have missed out on without timely intervention is why I have no hesitation to offer this option if there are clear signs and symptoms of problems.

If your child has severely crowded teeth, a lack of spacing between their baby teeth, or symptoms related to sleep disturbed breathing, bed wetting, or ear infections, be sure to talk to a dental professional who has experience with palate expansion as you're searching for various solutions.

MYOFUNCTIONAL THERAPY

I have referenced orofacial myofunctional therapy throughout this book. This chapter will finally delve deeper into this impactful therapy to help you understand which signs of poor airway health it can address, what is involved, and how to find the right therapist for your child and their needs.

Myofunctional therapy (MFT) involves creating awareness of improper patterns in the muscles of the mouth, face, and throat, and offers exercises to establish more normal patterns of breathing, chewing, swallowing, and speech. Before going into detail on MFT, I would like to share a patient story that will help highlight the ways in which this therapy can fill certain voids that other treatment methods cannot.

Case Study: 6.5-year-old requiring palate expansion

Jasmine is a patient of mine who I commenced palate expansion on at the age of six and a half years. Her parents were initially prompted to bring her in for an orthodontic consult. They described how she had problems with drooling and sleeping from birth. She started to see a speech therapist as a toddler, and they referred her to an ENT surgeon who suggested that removal of her adenoids and tonsils would help her sleep and speak better. The surgery did not resolve the speech issues, and she continued to breathe with her mouth open. Her sleep remained fragmented, there were concerns with attention, and by the afternoon she was overtired, leading to difficult behaviour.

I noted she had a very narrow (gutter) palate and narrow nasal floor and we commenced palate expansion – below are photos taken on the day expansion commenced, and at her 12-month review. The significant increase in palate vault width can offer exponential improvements in nasal airflow, plus more tongue space. Because of the severity of her narrow palate, treatment was impactful within weeks and her parents noted her tongue was fitting better in her mouth, she was closing her mouth more during sleep, sleeping more solidly, not waking as early (waking at 7am instead of 6am) and was less prone to tantrums and grumpiness. They remarked that, even with the plate in her mouth, she was pronouncing words clearer.

There is still an anterior open bite where the front upper and lower teeth don't meet. These are the result of an anterior tongue thrust or lowered posture of the tip of the tongue between her upper and lower teeth. It has closed significantly due to the improved space for the tongue to fit and function more normally within her mouth.

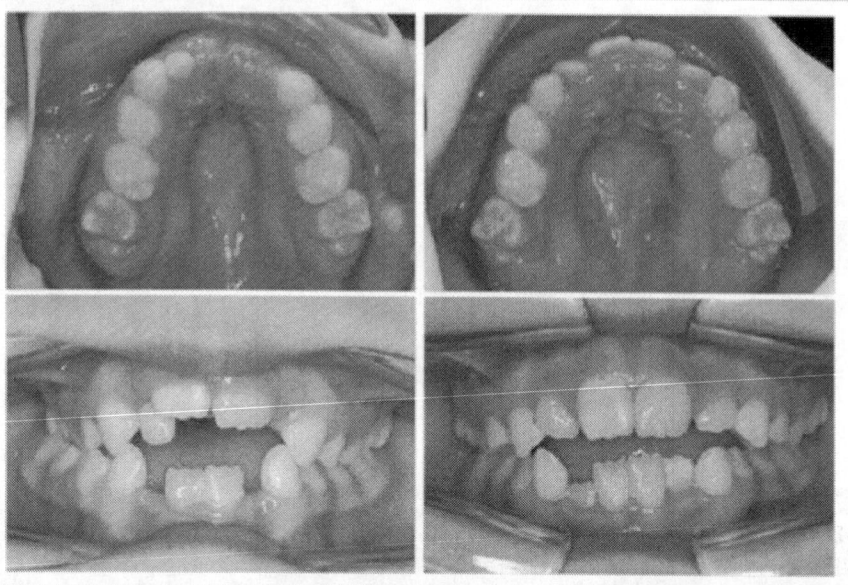

Despite the significant improvements and change for the whole family, there are still concerns of ADHD symptoms and she is on a waitlist to investigate this. I've shared prior that research tells us that, on average, children are at double the risk of inattention at age seven years if they mouth breathe, snore, or gasp during sleep at 30 months, even if they outgrow these symptoms.

There are missed opportunities for intervention. Poor structure of the palate reflects dysfunction of the oral and facial muscles. Remember, the first six years of life are critical for facial development, and we need to pay special attention to proper muscle stimulation during this period.

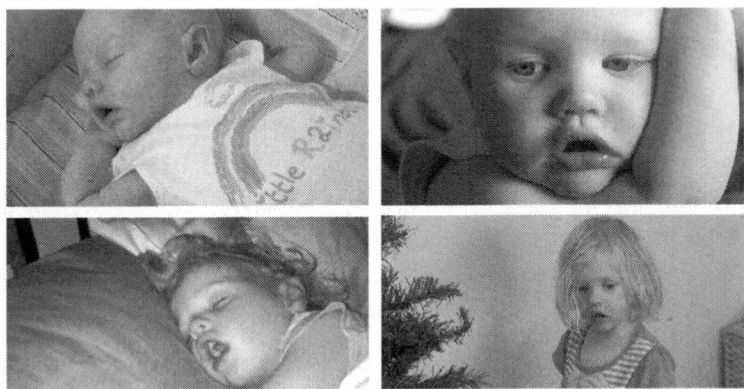

These are photos her mum supplied to me from when she was two months, 11 months, prior to her adenoid and tonsil surgery, and after her surgery. It is clear she had open mouth and low tongue posture at rest and low orofacial muscle tone even before she was born. After surgery, nasal disuse persisted. Since rest and sleep is where we spend most of the day, that is the best time frame to influence jaw development most.

While working with Jasmine, I identified an untreated posterior tongue-tie. Her functional history included breastfeeding for 18 months, but mum had recurrent mastitis (which could be related to poor tongue suction and drainage), while Jasmine was experiencing mouth breathing, snoring, gasping during sleep, fussy eating, problems with chewing and swallowing meat, and a tongue thrust or low tongue posture impacting speech. Her oral dysfunctions had compounded upon one another to the extent that performing the tongue-tie release would offer limited functional benefit unless more normal tongue tone, coordination, and patterns were established.

These dysfunctions of the mouth and face muscles not only affect jaw and airway development, but also airway function. When the tongue and throat muscles do not work well during the day, they will not work optimally for tongue to palate seal and keeping the airway open during sleep.

Now that Jasmine has completed both ENT surgery and palate expansion, we still need to address chronic nasal disuse and restore proper muscle tone, coordination, and function to ensure closed mouth nasal breathing and retrain new functional patterns.

In addition, although the bony expansion in the middle of her palate and nasal floor remodelling will be stable, the dental positions will not be – they will ultimately be determined by the balance between the tongue, lips, and cheeks. Without restoring normal tongue posture, lip seal, and nasal breathing, her teeth positions will be prone to relapse. This is where myofunctional therapy comes in.

One of the foundational goals of myofunctional therapy is to establish normal oral rest posture of the tongue, lips, and jaw through improving tone of the associated muscles.

We want to see good lip seal without strain, nasal breathing, and suction of the tongue to the palate at rest, including during sleep. Here, the back of the tongue can form a seal with the soft palate, effectively closing off the mouth breathing route and promoting nasal breathing. The suction also promotes the jaw to close in a relaxed position, and optimal tone and opening of the throat or airway muscles during sleep. This all leads to silent, slow, and effortless nasal breathing.

This resting tongue posture is also associated with the development of good swallowing and is the foundation for the development of good speech articulation.

The history of myofunctional therapy in the U.S. dates back to the early 1900s. The applications then were to help with tongue thrusts or lowered tongue posture and abnormal swallowing. It also aimed to improve orthodontic and speech problems. Now, it has become increasingly integrated into some orthodontic practices to help promote more normal facial growth and stability of results by addressing the underlying soft tissue causes of orthodontic problems.

Recently, attention has been mounting regarding the role of myofunctional therapy alongside other treatments in promoting nasal breathing and good upper airway muscle function in patients with snoring and OSA.[1-11] A meta-analysis published in the journal Sleep in 2015 by Camacho and co-workers pooled results of multiple studies and found that MFT could reduce OSA by an average of 50% in adults and 62% in children.[1] It is a very fast-growing area of research in sleep medicine. This is wonderful news for adults who need relief from this problem but are not able to tolerate other treatments or are reluctant to proceed with surgery.

Even better for you to understand as a parent is that the evidence suggests that it is most impactful in children and may play a critical role in stemming the development of later OSA. This is especially true when MFT is completed in combination with other interventions like tongue-tie release and palate expansion to restore normal tongue space and proper tongue mobility.

Oromyofunctional disorders (OMDs) refer to altered patterns of breathing, sucking, chewing, swallowing and speech, and oral rest posture. They all affect our throat or upper airway muscle function.

The alterations in muscle posture and tone play out most during sleep, when all the muscles are relaxed, and we are lying on our backs. Therefore, OMDs can be early warning signs for increased breathing dysfunction and unrestorative sleep down the track.

They have their origins in factors like tongue-ties, bottle feeding, overuse of pacifiers and sippy cups, allergies and mouth breathing, prematurity (low muscle tongue and use of nasogastric tubes), and soft diets. In other words, when some of the milestones discussed in the last section have been missed.

Common OMDs that may be addressed with myofunctional therapy include:

- open mouth breathing
- flaccid lips/poor lip seal
- reduced tongue mobility with tongue ties
- thumb sucking
- nail biting
- tongue thrusts and reverse swallows
- excessive drooling
- problems with chewing and swallowing
- speech misarticulations including lisps
- snoring and obstructive sleep apnoea
- persistent mouth breathing or snoring after removal of adenoids or tonsils
- teeth grinding during sleep
- eustachian tube dysfunction
- temporomandibular muscle pain and dysfunction
- orthodontic problems
- instability of orthodontic treatment results, and more

A common pattern I see are children who despite having gone through years of speech therapy, have seen little progress. They may be referred to my practice because a new speech therapist has identified a tongue-tie, or because the parents are concerned with mouth breathing, sleep, or orthodontic issues and we discover the speech concerns incidentally. The speech issues are merely an indication of a deeper-rooted issue, and we need to address the underlying poor muscle patterns. We do not treat speech as dental professionals, but parents often express how their child is speaking more clearly once we establish better muscle patterns with MFT.

MFT is most effective when implemented around the age of four or five at the earliest, when good compliance is possible. It involves working with a trained myofunctional therapist on a regular basis to gain awareness of optimal patterns, eliminate habits, and perform sequential exercises. These are tailored for each patient depending on their main patterns of dysfunction.

Once more normal rest posture is achieved, the next goals are to eliminate habits e.g., thumb sucking or nail biting, and then retrain normal chewing and swallowing.

The therapy is effective but relies heavily on patient compliance with daily exercises. For young children, this will depend on a good rapport with the therapist and commitment from parents to become the 'therapist' at home to motivate them.

MFT often requires collaboration with allergists and ENT specialists to ensure a clear nasal airway, as well as with dental professionals to ensure the jaw structures are of sufficient size and position to allow proper tongue placement. It is also important that children are assessed for tongue-ties

The end goal is habituation or incorporating new habits into the daily routine and activities. Constant repetition provides sensory input to the somatosensory cortex of the brain, creating new neural pathways so these habits become automatic. The more frequent the input, the more efficiently these patterns can be incorporated into sleep. Prolonged, continuous training is better than brief intermittent periods of practice over time. Brain neuroplasticity, or the ability to re-organize and form new neural connections, is usually highest in childhood, making it easier for these practices to stick.

In our practice, initial appointments will be more frequent, occurring every two weeks, and will then be gradually reduced in frequency with the expectation that activities are continued at home – often for a year – to cement the new habits.

The biggest downfall with myofunctional therapy is its reliance on compliance; it is often difficult for busy parents and children to incorporate it into their lives. For this reason, I will often introduce habit correcting devices like Healthy Start Habit Correctors to help correct muscle balance and improve tongue posture whilst children spend time watching TV or reading.

Myofunctional therapists most commonly have a background in either speech and language pathology or dental therapy. Speech pathologists first developed an interest because chronic open mouth breathing resulted in muscle patterns associated with speech articulation issues. In Brazil, every speech and language therapist receives training in myofunctional therapy.

Becoming a myofunctional therapist requires completion of a 28-hour introductory program. The best results are going to come from a therapist who has completed multiple additional courses, and who has also completed multiple professional development courses in the areas of tongue-ties, sleep, and airway health. Experience in this area is critical to ensuring the most targeted exercises and best progress for your child.

It is important to check your therapist's credentials, experience, and the feedback they have received from other professionals they collaborate with. You should also, of course, be happy with the relationship you and your child develop with them.

Case Study: Myofunctional therapy and Myobrace appliance for 8-year-old with orthodontic concerns

One of our patient's school dental services had suggested an orthodontic consultation to discuss intervention for her 'overbite' or flared front teeth. She had a history of thumb sucking and had developed a pattern of atypical swallowing. A tongue tie was identified, as was lowered tongue resting posture, and she commenced myofunctional therapy to repattern normal resting tongue posture and lip seal and to promote nasal breathing.

The tongue-tie was released during the treatment to achieve those aims, including more tongue-to-palate contact at the back half of the tongue. She also used a Myobrace, a myofunctional training device, for one hour per day and during sleep to reinforce new muscle habits. These results – achieved within a few months – demonstrate that, by controlling the orofacial muscles, a new equilibrium zone was achieved for the teeth, and they were able to move into alignment without the use of braces. She has achieved a broader arch and fuller smile. She no longer rests her lower lip under the upper teeth, which would have worsened the overjet if left unchecked for years.

Compared to a mechanical approach, this is a more stable result. If the patient maintains awareness and continues reinforcing new patterns, it is likely she will not require braces as her adult teeth come through.

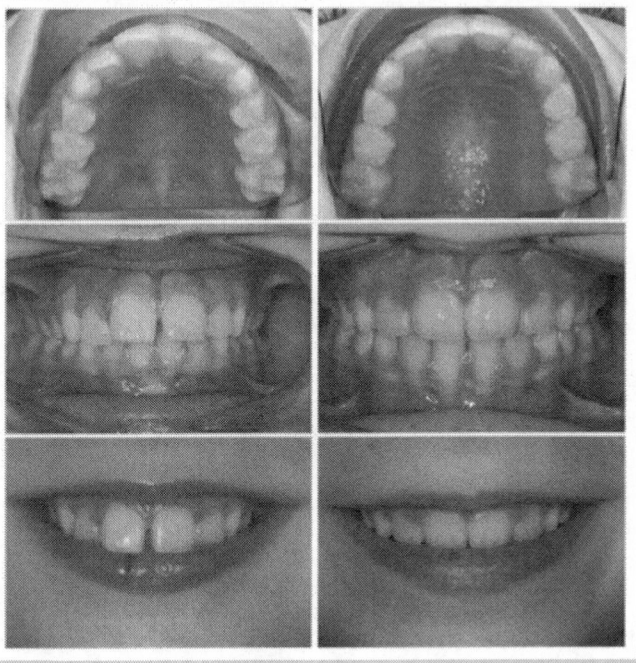

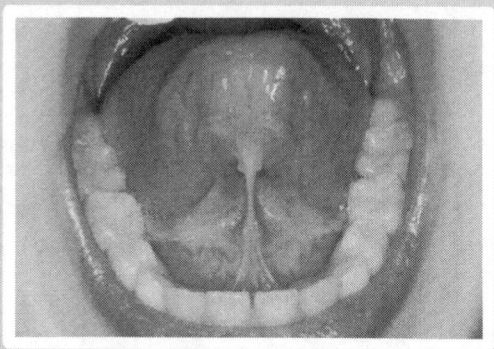

Case Study: Myofunctional therapy for 6-year-old with tongue-tie and mouth breathing

This six-year-old girl originally presented to me with her mother who had concerns about overcrowding of her mouth and the appearance of lower "shark teeth." She decided to see me for a second orthodontic opinion, as she was aware there was a tongue-tie, and she wanted my input on this at the same time.

Her functional history included:
* Born premature – 35 weeks, nasogastric tube fed (NGT) for three days
* Emergency c-section, torticollis
* Breastfed for 24 months; slow weight gain – "failure to thrive" from months nine to twelve
* Suspected silent reflux
* Allergies – eczema, anaphylactic to nuts and sesame seeds, and cat and dog hair
* Nail biting
* Regular headaches, regular chiropractor to release neck tension
* Audible breathing during sleep linked to allergies
* Restlessness during sleep
* Tired during the day and after school

The big thing that stood out to me was that she was mouth breathing. I noticed Grade 2 tonsils and that she could breathe comfortably through her nose when asked to keep her mouth closed for two minutes. I suggested myofunctional therapy was a good front line option for her to reinforce nasal breathing.

After four sessions of therapy in preparation for tongue tie release, she stated in her own words that she was sleeping better and eating better. She was not waking up as much during the night and was waking up later in the morning. She felt her breathing made her feel more relaxed. She felt like she was able to chew better and could eat more different foods – for example, prior to treatment, she was unable to eat cheese, but was able to after treatment. She was using a Myomunchee appliance for chewing practice and found that this helped her lips stay together more whilst chewing.

Three weeks post-tongue tie release, her mum reported:

- Less picky eating - now eating meat. Before, she had to provide a different meal from the rest of the family with all the foods separated, and now she could eat with everyone.
- More energy.
- Happier and more confident in her abilities.
- Chiropractor reports significant release of neck tension.
- Patient perceives her neck feels freer. Feels more flexible during gymnastics and can move her feet more easily during jazz dance.
- Currently taking antihistamines with the onset of hay fever season, but it was remarkable that she did not have to do this for a six-week period during therapy.
- The absence of headaches has persisted.

At the 18-month mark I checked in with mum to see how things were going and, looking back on everything, what she considered to be the biggest impact for her daughter.

She said that firstly there was no more intense teeth grinding that could be heard in another room. This is good news, as teeth grinding is a strong red flag indicating disturbed breathing during sleep. Secondly, she was putting on weight and rounding out well. As a premature baby who had been failing to thrive, it was a relief to see her catch up in size to her peers.

This case study highlights that the muscles of the mouth and throat are important for so many vital functions, and when one is not functioning right it is not unusual for it to impact multiple areas of a child's development – including their sleep and breathing. A parent may come in with one concern and be surprised to find that many other aspects are changed positively with this intervention.

The key take-home message here is not to overlook this non-invasive therapy to help restore more normal function. Even after surgery or orthodontic treatment, remember that MFT could be the critical missing link to address the root causes of problems and restore healthy oral rest posture, nasal breathing and promote more normal jaw and airway development.

11

AIRWAY HEALTH IN ADULTHOOD

As parents, we always put our children first. I hope that, through all the preceding chapters, I've been able to guide you through the steps of solving your child's problems or being proactive to help them achieve better breathing for life.

But this chapter is all about you and your adult loved ones. Perhaps you picked up this book wanting to find a path to help your child avoid airway issues that you or your partner are currently experiencing. Or maybe you wanted to be proactive for your child and have since recognised symptoms in yourself or other friends or family that may be related to hidden airway problems.

I'd like to equip you with all the information you need to recognise problems and ensure your own breathing and airway health is optimized. I hope to see you possess the greatest vitality to raise your children and enjoy them most while staving off chronic diseases so you can enjoy and actively contribute to the lives of your grandchildren and even great grandchildren too!

In addition, if you're planning for another child, it may be a good time to spare a thought about airway health during pregnancy. Due to things like hormone changes, weight gain and more, pregnancy is a time when we are very vulnerable to sleep disturbed breathing, and this is linked to increased risk of high blood pressure, gestational diabetes, pre-eclampsia, intra-uterine growth restriction, and pre-term births.[1] Optimizing sleep and breathing even before falling pregnant is where the future of airway health and the best start to life begins.

When I first became qualified in dental sleep medicine, there was often a one-size-fits-all approach to managing adult airway problems. This mainly involved dealing with the night-time symptoms of restricted airways with CPAP. Dental appliances were largely reserved as the backup solution. More recently, there has been a shift to more precise and personalized options which is hugely promising for patients.

This means there is an increasing array of options that can be offered and combined to target individual risk factors, minimize unwanted side effects, maximize comfort, and match personal preferences.

For adult patients, the future is beyond relying on band-aid solutions to address symptoms of poor breathing during sleep. There is a growing focus on restoring normal airway structure and function, including new approaches to address poor jaw structures, and interventions to improve nasal breathing and muscle function. These offer a path to not only reclaim the full restorative benefits of sleep, but to restore airway health, and in turn general health and wellness.

The increasing array of targeted options is great news, as one of the most common barriers for people investigating sleep disturbed breathing is that they don't see themselves being able to use the traditional treatment options for the rest of their lives.

The first step is recognizing the scope of the airway problems in adults. Here are some of the common warning signs – many of which are similar to what you may see in children.

Night-time symptoms include:

- mouth breathing
- snoring
- pauses in breathing or waking gasping for air
- teeth grinding
- unexplained awakenings
- nocturia (the frequent need to urinate in the middle of sleep)
- night-time sweating
- difficulty falling asleep

Daytime symptoms include:

- feeling unrefreshed on waking
- unexplained daytime tiredness or dragging through the day
- excessive daytime sleepiness
- morning headaches
- mood swings and feelings of depression
- difficulty concentrating or memory problems
- decreased libido
- high blood pressure

These days, many dentists are trained to identify the warning signs in the mouth that are linked to increased risk, and they can be good people to consult with during your regular dental visits. Otherwise, you can seek a consultation with your general medical practitioner.

The next step is usually a sleep study but as we mentioned with children, if we are focused on airway health and achieving optimal sleep and breathing, we need to look beyond OSA and recognise the more subtle precursor forms of airway problems such as mouth breathing, snoring, and UARS.

UPPER AIRWAY RESISTANCE SYNDROME

I want to review Upper Airway Resistance Syndrome (UARS) here because as parents of young children, many of you will fall into the groups of slimmer individuals and premenopausal women.

Prior to menopause, progesterone makes the dilator muscles of the throat more active and offers some protection against the prolonged airway collapses that define OSA. This is why until menopause, women are less affected by OSA than men.

This group is more likely to have UARS or increased efforts to breathe at the first signs of restricted airflow. This is associated with arousals from sleep, and people who suffer from this don't get the deep restorative sleep that makes them feel refreshed.

Dr Steven Parks, an Ear, Nose and Throat (ENT) specialist and author of the book "Sleep Interrupted: A physician reveals the #1 reason why so many of us are sick and tired" describes UARS as being responsible for an epidemic of fatigue in the US.[2]

In adults, this condition is linked to chronic stress and common medical ailments and problems like teeth grinding, TMD (temporomandibular joint disorder) and jaw muscle pain, headaches, insomnia, and anxiety disorders. Breathing problems are often not considered when these conditions are diagnosed.

Although UARS is more common than OSA, it tends to go unrecognised and unaddressed.[3] Due to the focus on OSA, some people are told they don't have breathing issues, and the conditions they suffer with become accepted as their "normal."

But apart from the signs and symptoms above, the mouth leaves clues. The single most important risk factor for UARS is a small mouth. Generally, these people do not have a problem of excess weight or fat in the throat or tongue. The jaw may be narrow or retruded, and there may be a history of extractions of premolar teeth to relieve dental crowding that occurred due to jaw underdevelopment.

If the tongue is disproportionately large, it will be prone to falling back into the throat and blocking the airway during sleep. Those who suffer will often not sleep on their backs. They prefer side or stomach sleeping. Stomach sleeping may be a compensation to keep breathing and can raise a red flag.

Some will complain of rhinitis or sinus problems, which can be traced back to narrow palates that form the floor of the nose and sinus passages.

Patients most commonly have some form of fatigue or excessive daytime sleepiness that may be masked with the intake of coffee or regular exercise.

Some may say they have vivid dreams because they are waking frequently during their dreams and can recall them. The REM phase of sleep – where dreaming occurs – is also the phase where the airway muscles have reduced tone and are most vulnerable to collapse. Some will not remember dreams because they never enter this deeper phase of sleep in the first place.

Due to the constant dumping of stress hormones into the body, patients may have sleep onset or sleep maintenance insomnia. They may not be able to get to sleep, or if they wake – typically around the 3 a.m. REM sleep phase – they may find it difficult to get back to sleep.

One study has shown that nearly a quarter of people with UARS will have low blood pressure. They may also present with cold hands and feet.

Ready for 'fight or flight'

The autonomic nervous system regulates the body's unconscious functions such as breathing, digestion, heart rate, and blood pressure. It's divided into the sympathetic nervous system (SNS) – which activates the fight or flight response and mobilises the blood flow and energy for any challenges – and the parasympathetic nervous system (PNS) – which is involved more with 'rest and digest' or 'feed and breed' activities that occur at rest, especially after a meal.

In UARS patients, the nervous system is very responsive to the threat of airway collapse compared to those with OSA. This chronic low-grade stress night after night, year after year, tips the balance in favour of sympathetic nervous system activation. This activates what is called the Hypothalamic–Pituitary–Adrenal (HPA) axis, causing a cascade of hormones which ultimately results in an increase in cortisol, the body's main stress hormone.

Normally when danger has passed, cortisol levels calm down and the heart, blood pressure, and the body's systems should return to normal. However, in the presence of the constant threat to breathing, the body's alarm system remains on high alert and these hormones can result in anxiety and depression, high blood pressure, and heart disease.

Blood gets shifted away from the gastrointestinal system to the heart muscles at the expense of proper digestion, and symptoms like chronic diarrhea, constipation, indigestion, chronic bloating, and reflux can appear.

There may also be some association with problems with sexual function like polycystic ovaries and erectile dysfunction.

Central sensitisation syndromes and anxiety disorders

When the nervous system is in a constant high state of reactivity, central sensitisation may occur.[4-8] Pain receptors are sensitised to stimuli that in normal circumstances would not cause pain. It can be likened to being on edge during a scary movie. Someone could tap you on the back and make you jump because of the heightened state you are in.

Central sensitisation or functional somatic syndromes are a group of conditions that present with symptoms like pain and fatigue that seem out of proportion to any identifiable pathology. Not everyone with UARS will have these, but there are now several experts linking these conditions and treatment of the airway to reduced symptoms. This highlights the need for sleep breathing problems to be considered when these syndromes are present. These may include:

- Chronic fatigue syndrome
- Fibromyalgia
- Migraine/tension headache syndrome
- Irritable bowel syndrome
- Temporomandibular syndrome
- Multiple chemical sensitivities
- Anxiety disorders – including panic disorder, generalised anxiety disorder, and post-traumatic stress disorder

These conditions tend to be linked to milder forms of sleep breathing disturbances and are less common as the severity of OSA increases.

Many of these syndromes have very non-specific symptoms. For example, consider chronic fatigue syndrome. The most common symptom is fatigue severe enough to interfere with daily activities that has been present for six months. To get a diagnosis, a person must have at least four of the following symptoms:

- Loss of memory or poor concentration
- Feeling unrefreshed after a night's sleep
- Chronic insomnia
- Muscle pain
- Frequent headaches
- Multiple instances of joint pain without redness or swelling

- Frequent sore throat or tender and swollen lymph nodes in the neck and armpit.

There are no lab tests that can be done to screen for this condition, and it is a challenging diagnosis. Many of these symptoms are common to sleep disturbed breathing.

The great news is that Dr Avram Gold has shown that the same treatments that are offered for patients with OSA to improve airflow can improve symptoms of a wide range of functional somatic syndromes.[9-10]

Teeth grinding: a marker of airway dysfunction

One of the most common problems we encounter as dentists is jaw muscle pain suffered by people who wake up grinding their teeth. They may complain of tension-type or migraine headaches.

The traditional option for these patients is a dental splint or plastic appliance that sits between their upper and lower teeth to protect them from wearing down. These have not been proven to reduce teeth grinding activity in the long term and are another example of how modern medicine and dentistry focus on managing symptoms rather than addressing root causes.

The research now suggests that teeth grinding is often associated with arousals from sleep and is likely a compensation to recruit the muscles to keep the airway open.[11-13]

This may offer some protection against OSA or the more severe collapses and blockages of the airway.

Australian dentist Dr Nischal Singh completed a prize-winning research project that investigated the degree of tooth wear in baby teeth alongside breathing in sleep study results.[14] While there was no correlation with OSA, there seemed to be a relationship with the milder breathing disturbances seen in UARS. This seems consistent with the hypothesis that teeth grinding may have a protective role in preventing full-blown apnoeas.

One of the problems we are starting to appreciate in dentistry is that increasing the space between the upper and lower jaws without repositioning the lower jaw forward results in the lower jaw and tongue rotating backward and impinging on the airway space. Lavigne and team conducted a study which demonstrated that 60% of patients who were given a night guard for sleep grinding had an aggravation of breathing during sleep.[15] So the common practice of issuing these appliances for patients grinding their teeth could be worsening their breathing. It also helps explain why many patients report they seem to find the appliance by the side of the bed in the morning.

The American College of Prosthodontists – the specialty of dentistry most concerned with managing the problem of tooth wear – released a statement in 2016 which said that a history of sleep must be taken before offering a guard for night-time grinding.[16] This means that before you get a night-time splint for teeth grinding, make sure your dentist has ruled out airway problems.

COMBATING POOR AIRWAY HEALTH AS AN ADULT

This section provides an overview of the various options available to adults with dysfunctional airways and disturbed sleep breathing.

While we do have more individualised means of treatment than we used to, there is still a need for greater integrative team care to ensure that patients have access to those solutions that serve them and their lifestyles best.

Some of the options are most helpful to minimise symptoms during sleep. But, as with children, restoring nasal breathing and proper tongue function and jaw structures should be the ultimate end goal for long term stability of results and optimal health and wellness.

In children, it's possible to modify the jaw structures with orthodontic intervention to secure a better trajectory of breathing for life and avoid problems developing in adulthood. However, in adults, you will understand the growing role that jaw surgeries have when we miss the chance to get things going early.

Conservative options

In mild cases, conservative options such as weight loss, reducing alcohol, sleeping on one's side, and the use of nasal sprays may be helpful to relieve symptoms. Myofunctional therapy also has an important role in restoring wellness for adults, especially in conjunction with other front-line options.

Weight loss. With increased weight gain, fat starts to accumulate in the walls of the throat and base of the tongue, compounding the problem of a structurally narrow airway prone to collapsing.

The Wisconsin Sleep Cohort study demonstrated that a 10% reduction in body weight could predict a 25% decrease in AHI.[17] At the same time, a 10% increase in body weight predicted a 32% increase in AHI or increased the odds of developing moderate to severe OSA in four years by four to six times.

Lifestyle modification to reduce weight can be difficult. Poor sleep can disrupt hormones, including those that control appetite like elevated ghrelin (which signals hunger) and reduced leptin (which signals feeling full). In addition, excessive daytime sleepiness and lethargy can make it difficult for a person to exercise and they may be more prone to unhealthy eating. It creates a perfect storm for obesity and a whole cascade of metabolic problems that increase the risk of cardiovascular disease and diabetes. This perpetuates the cycle of breathing and metabolic problems.

It's been my experience that front-line options to address a poor airway can help people find the energy and motivation to be more active and shed weight easier. Those with a high BMI are more likely to benefit from bariatric surgery.

Reducing alcohol. Alcohol is a known muscle relaxant, and this will impact the tongue and muscles that keep the airway open. It is best to avoid this before bed.

Positional therapy. When the tongue does not rest properly suctioned to the palate, it is more likely to sit low and obstruct the throat in back sleepers. Positional therapy aims to get people sleeping on their side instead and may include strapping a tennis ball to the patient's back, or a wearable device that vibrates when it detects the patient lying on their back to prompt them to change position. These tactics can help reduce obstruction of the airway and may be helpful for people who have airway collapses only when sleeping on their backs. However, many people may find it difficult or uncomfortable to control their sleeping position.

Nasal sprays. Sprays can help reduce swelling and inflammation in the airway and make it easier to breathe through the nose. With reduced resistance to nasal airflow, breathing is smoother, and inhaling will no longer result in so many of the vacuum pressures responsible for the collapse of the airway.

Myofunctional therapy. We've discussed myofunctional therapy in great detail in Chapter 10. In summary, growing research has supported it as an important intervention to restore nasal breathing and normal tongue tone, and as an effective adjunct to other front-line options to alleviate snoring and OSA.

Case Study: Myofunctional therapy and tongue tie release for adult female with speech concerns

This case study highlights how myofunctional therapy can help improve sleep and airway health in conjunction with tongue-tie release to facilitate better tongue mobility.

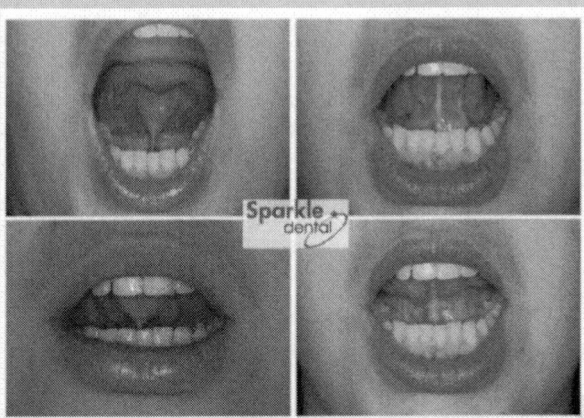

Before and after tongue-tie release

The main prompt for the initial assessment was the patient's desire to gain more freedom of movement of her tongue. She was a singer who had been working with speech therapists for over a year to get her "r" sounds. She was confident the tongue-tie was not affecting her speech but wanted more assistance prior to a foreign language performance. She had also noticed that she was often waking in the morning with a sore tongue from biting on it in her sleep.

Other symptoms reported during the initial consult included:
- some difficulty swallowing tablets
- monthly headaches: lasting half a day, associated with aura – restricted vision for the rest of the day
- chronic dull ache in neck and shoulder area – releases do not hold following massage, so she had just gotten used to it
- unrestorative sleep: adequate sleep time but was waking feeling exhausted, hard to get out of bed – could stay in bed for another couple of hours if nothing to do, may take a nap in the afternoon
- was sometimes taking three to four hours to fall asleep
- mouth breathing and husband reported snoring
- aware of jaw clenching
- periods of sore joints (wrists and elbows) which could wake her up

Severe restriction of tongue mobility was confirmed. I suggested that, due to a constricted palate and lack of optimal tongue space, I would offer a partial tongue-tie release to improve tongue mobility if she had a good response to the therapy. Releasing the entire tongue tie in a mouth without adequate tongue space could potentially aggravate sleep breathing issues further.

Observations over five months of myofunctional therapy prior to tongue tie release (prolonged due to Covid-19 restrictions on elective treatment) were as follows:
- Swallowing tablets was easier
- No more aura associated with headaches
- Tongue biting and sore tongue eliminated
- Less clenching
- No soreness in wrists and elbows

During the height of Covid-19, she stopped exercises for a while and the clenching, jaw pain, and sore joints returned, but she resumed exercises and found relief again. She perceived the sore joints to be part of a stress response.

One week review post tongue tie release:
- "R" sounds had become easier
- Was waking up feeling more refreshed – not so heavy in the morning, not feeling like she couldn't move
- Tongue naturally lifting to roof of the mouth – after day three

Two-month review post tongue tie release:
- All prior improvements had held
- Noticed that the "R" sounds were coming in very easily during singing.
- Perceived the tongue as too big for the back of her mouth but sleeping and breathing much better
- More energy – started going to gym two to three times per week
- Reported she had had severe depression and been seeing a psychologist for the past 10 years but felt particularly good for the past two months and the psychologist told her there was no need for further visits
- Overall was feeling happy in life

Frontline options

In moderate or severe cases, or where symptoms are affecting daily function, frontline treatments can generally be classified into CPAP, oral appliances, and surgery.

In general, options like CPAP and oral appliances tend to be helpful to improve symptoms and breathing during sleep. Surgery offers a variety of targeted options that can help get you on your way to restoring airway structure and function day and night, without the reliance on daily compliance.

Continuous positive airway pressure. In adults, the standard treatment option is continuous positive airway pressure (CPAP). A mask is worn over the nose or face and is connected by a hose to a toaster-sized device that delivers air into the airway. It essentially works like a reverse vacuum cleaner, blowing air into the airway to help prop it open during breathing.

Many studies have proven that it reduces obstructive breathing events and the negative health impacts of many medical conditions.

However, the main problem is that relatively few people can tolerate it. For example, it is generally accepted that up to 30% of people can't tolerate it after diagnosis, and, of those who can, fewer than 50% will be able to continue using it in the long term.

Even those that use it are considered 'adherent' if they can wear it at least four hours a night. This is typically the first half of the night, but most often it is the second half of the night when people enter the deepest, most restorative phase of sleep and are likely to have the most breathing disturbances. This reduces its overall effectiveness in resolving symptoms and consequences. The main challenges with people using CPAP are:

- skin irritation or discomfort from the mask
- claustrophobia, nasal congestion
- transient insomnia
- dry mouth
- aerophagia or swallowing of air, causing symptoms like reflux, belching, flatulence, cramping, and abdominal discomfort

Based on growing evidence to support their use, oral appliances have emerged as the leading alternative to CPAP for mild sleep apnoea – or in more severe cases, when CPAP therapy is refused or is not tolerated.

Mandibular advancement devices. These dental appliances, also worn during sleep, help position the lower jaw forward. This pulls the base of the tongue forward (since it is attached to the lower jaw) and prevents it from falling back into a collapsed airway. This position also increases tension of the upper dilator muscles of the airway in the region behind the soft palate and tongue. This helps reduce collapsibility of the airway to keep it open.

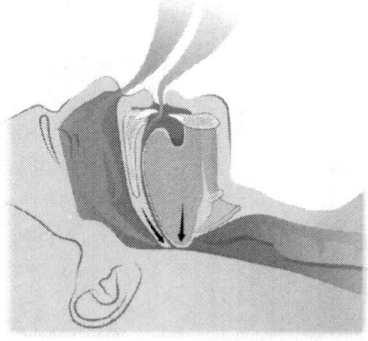 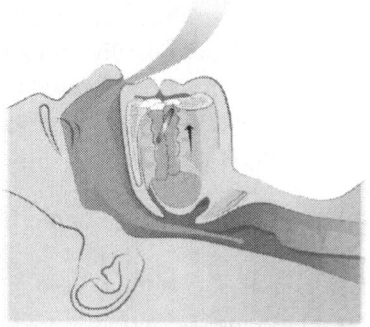

Most studies comparing oral appliances with CPAP have found that CPAP is more effective at reducing sleep disturbed breathing and achieving complete control of OSA.[18]

However, due to poor compliance with CPAP and the better adherence to wearing an oral appliance, research has shown that in an average patient, both will have similar clinical effectiveness in terms of improving health outcomes like reducing excessive day sleepiness and improving blood pressure and quality of life.

The degree of reduction tends to vary among different people. The predictors of success are younger age, lower body mass, smaller neck circumference, and being female.

There are many different designs of oral appliances and no one design has been proven to be most effective. However the cheaper 'boil and bite' appliances that are mouldable when immersed in hot water are less effective, as they tend to be bulkier and more difficult to tolerate. Custom-fitted appliances provided by qualified dentists who have training in this field are the superior option.

The main issue with long-term use of oral appliances has to do with changes in the way the teeth bite together. This can be expected because the teeth are used as anchors to move the lower jaw. Many dentists become concerned with this, but it is often not discernible by patients. Even when it is, most perceive this as a negligible price to pay for a better night's sleep and greater capacity to function during the day.

Sleep surgery. CPAP and MADs are band-aid solutions that patients must rely on every night. They help reduce symptoms of poor breathing when used during sleep, but don't do anything to help patients restore better airway function to wean themselves off treatment, nor are they particularly well targeted.

In contrast, sleep surgery offers an array of options that can be personalised and precisely targeted to each individual's sites of airway restriction, plus a means to unlock missed developmental milestones in childhood to restore both normal structure and function of the airway. This offers an alternative for patients who want to work towards optimal health rather than just managing night-time symptoms. It's a means to ensure that people can breathe well through their nose with their mouth closed – the way nature intended us to. For adults, sleep surgery can also be used to:

- address excess soft tissue in the airway at the level of the nose, soft palate, or tongue base
- remodel the structural support of the airway through expanding the palate and advancing the jaws
- address poor tongue tone through a newer intervention called Upper Airway Stimulation

Rather than one surgery being completely effective for all individuals, the surgery should be matched to each person's specific pattern or sites of blockage. The idea is to customise and combine surgeries and look at the overall success for each person.

One of the problems that can occur in sleep surgery is compartmentalisation. For example, an Ear Nose and Throat (ENT) surgeon may look down the airway with a nasoendoscope (a camera on a flexible tube that is inserted down the throat through the nose) and focus on the excess tissues inside the airway. But not considering the outer frame of the airway (the jaws) is comparable to "tunnel vision."

In the past, this has led to a more **resective approach** to sleep surgery – reducing long soft palates or parts of the base of the tongue that are collapsing into the throat. Now there is a greater appreciation that these excessive tissues may be disproportionately large due to deficient bony skeleton support.

Another approach is to **expand or advance the jaws or 'airway box.'** This involves skeletal or jaw surgery, which is most often performed by a Maxillofacial Surgeon.

Integrating these two fields of surgery is key to the most effective and conservative procedures for each patient.

In addition, the dynamics of the airway during sleep need to be considered – and the way air is flowing can change the patterns of airway collapse in each patient. Rather than just a scope or looking at jaw structures on an x-ray, drug induced sedation endoscopy (DISE) – or viewing the airway with a scope or video camera whilst a person is under drug-induced sleep – can offer greater clues on how to treat a patient.

It's not enough to make structures wider – the end goal must be to promote better stability and function, including the restoration of nasal breathing and good muscle tone.

MMA surgery or double jaw advancement surgery. Maxillomandibular advancement surgery (MMA) is regarded as the most effective surgery for OSA, short of a tracheostomy or inserting a tube into the windpipe through an incision at the front of the neck.

MMA surgery involves advancing both the upper and lower jaws forward in the face. This advancement increases airway tension, gives more space for the tongue to sit properly without encroaching upon the throat or airway space, and provides more airway volume for all the soft tissues to fit. The net effect is reduced airway collapsibility during inspiration.

It is considered a multi-level surgery because it addresses multiple sites at risk of obstruction, including the soft palate, tongue base, and lateral or side walls of the airway.

It is to be expected that the soft palate and tongue base may be at increased risk of collapse due to gravity when sleeping on the back during sleep. The collapse of the side walls of the throat that connect the soft palate and tongue base is associated with more severe OSA and is most strongly associated with greater deficiency of jaw development and skeletal support of the airway. This may warrant more aggressive treatment including MMA due to increased risk of future cardiovascular complications.

MMA has been shown to significantly improve breathing and sleep parameters measured on overnight sleep studies, subjective sleep symptoms, quality of life scores, diastolic blood pressure, and neurocognitive testing scores.[20-21] It has also been effective in patients with obesity and severe OSA.

The average hospitalisation time of MMA surgery is less than a week, with most patients returning to work within four to ten weeks post-surgery.

However, MMA is the most invasive surgery with relatively higher risks. For this reason, except for people with very severe OSA of facial imbalances they want to address, it is largely considered a 'Stage 2' surgery, after more conservative 'Stage 1' surgeries that precisely target individual risk factors like the nose, soft palate, or tongue.

Case Study: Maxillomandibular Advancement (MMA) Surgery

At the time of his MMA surgery and treatment by Drs Robert Riley and Audrey Yoon at Stanford Medical Centre, Mick was 48 years old with a long history of allergies and breathing problems tracing back to his childhood. He was finding he couldn't fight his tiredness or compensate for his short-term memory like he could when he was younger. He described how compensating led to a cycle of his body being in complete stress mode – he couldn't sleep well and put on 30 pounds of weight, which only worsened his breathing and sleep. He was finding himself falling asleep at the wheel of his car almost daily and waking only to the beeps of the horn from other drivers. His sleep study found an AHI of 80, or an average of 80 obstructive events lasting 10 seconds or more every hour of sleep.

Mick had previously trialled CPAP, had soft palate surgery and a genioglossus advancement (which had offered improvement for 10 years), as well as a dental appliance.

His sleep surgeon, Dr Rob Riley, suggested MMA surgery. Although a frightening prospect, Dr Riley had also suggested that if he didn't do it, Mick would likely be dead within five years from a car accident or heart attack. Mick was getting married and had a young stepdaughter he wanted to be around for. He opted for the surgery.

The following photos demonstrate the changes in his facial balance, tongue and airway space, and the volume of his airway before and after surgery.

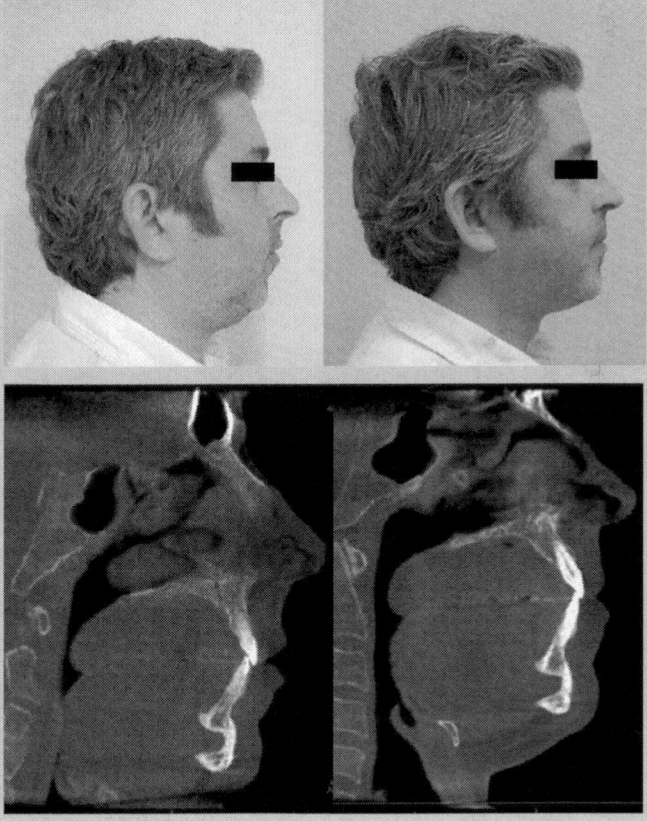

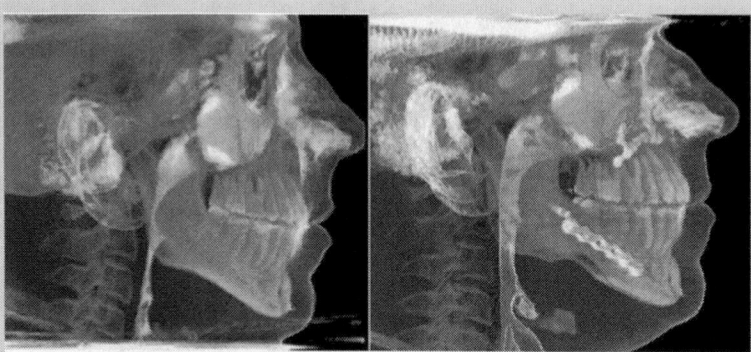

Case photos shared and used with permission by Dr Audrey Yoon

When I interviewed Mick about his experience, he had lost further weight and had a much more youthful appearance.

Mick was overall very happy with his experience:
- He almost never snored. His wife had reported a couple of occasions he did which were related to allergies.
- His short-term memory had improved.
- He didn't fall asleep in the car anymore.
- He had lost a lot of weight.

He did experience significant side effects, including:
- For the first three years post-surgery, he could not look at himself in the mirror or in photos because he could not recognise who he saw. It was only in the past few months that he had become more accustomed to his reflection and began feeling comfortable with his new look. This was something he did not feel adequately prepared for compared to risks of numbness and infection.
- He now has ongoing numbness of his lower right lip and chin, which he was fully aware was a risk of the procedure. While he has full motor function, it means he must drink with a straw rather than from a glass, to avoid spilling.
- He also ensures he wipes his mouth after each bite because he can't feel what remains on his face.

Overall, he felt these side effects were a small price to pay for his new lease on life.

From a parent's perspective, what is interesting to know about this case is that the clues and opportunities to intervene were present very early on. Mick identified himself as a child that had a lot of allergies. He had his adenoids and tonsils taken out around the age of 10 years. This is a relatively late age for this operation and is well past the age that we would normally expect adenoids and tonsils to start receding. This means it is most likely he had an obstructive airway and persistent mouth breathing whilst his facial structures were growing. This led to a vertical growth pattern, with the lower jaw swinging down and back. It is subclinical and not well recognised. The key to optimal wellness is to help children's faces grow forward.

Phase 1 or site-specific surgeries. While MMA is highly effective, it is not without significant risk, and some people may be treated with more targeted and less invasive options. The Stanford Sleep Surgery Protocol suggests more site-specific, or Stage 1, surgeries be considered in the first instance to see if MMA can be avoided.[22-24]

The main targets for Stage 1 surgery are the nose, the soft palate, and the tongue. I will focus on helping you understand the emerging role of adult expansion surgery to address nasal obstruction and more.

Nasal surgery

When it comes to OSA management, nasal breathing is too often overlooked. And yet, if there is nasal obstruction, other frontline therapies such as CPAP and MAD will not be as effective.

Any obstruction of the nose increases resistance to nasal airflow. This resistance during inspiration makes the airway more susceptible to collapsing.

Traditionally, an ENT surgeon would use a scope to look inside the nose for deviated nasal septums, swollen nasal turbinates, poor nasal valve function, and enlarged adenoids. Intra-nasal surgery would address these areas.

In my practice, I see patients who have had nasal or sinus surgery but didn't find that it made a difference for their symptoms of nasal obstruction or OSA, and they are then referred to me to explore oral appliance therapy. It is not uncommon for nasal surgery to yield disappointing results.

Researchers at Stanford Medical Centre did a retrospective analysis of patients with persistent nasal obstruction following nasal surgery.[25] They found that this was associated with having a narrow, high arch palate. In other words, the patients had a narrow nasal floor or smaller nasal box, which is why it wasn't as effective. This team proposed those patients would benefit from nasal floor remodelling procedures such as adult palate expansion surgery.

Adult palate expansion

The narrow, high-arch palate has been increasingly recognised as a significant risk factor in the development of OSA.

Narrow, high-arch palates signal narrow nasal floors, reduced nasal airway volumes, increased resistance to nasal airflow, and increased risk of airway collapse when inspiring during sleep. They also reduce space for the tongue to fit and maintain good tongue-to-palate contact that keeps the upper airway open.

The narrow hard palate also reduces structural support for the soft palate, which attaches to it. Elongated soft palate, itself a risk factor for OSA, has been associated with narrow, high-arch palates.

Expanding the palate can be an impactful option to improve airflow in the nose, and at the level of the soft palate, and base of the tongue, as opposed to resecting tissues inside the airway at these regions.

As we've discussed, palate expansion in children has been very well established to improve the nasal airway and help reduce OSA. An orthodontic device is supported by the teeth with a screw in the middle. As this screw is turned by parents, it applies a widening force across the mid-palate suture. The two halves of the palate are gradually separated, and new bone forms in a process called 'distraction osteogenesis.' This widens the palate at the area of the nasal floor.

It was previously not thought possible to achieve the same outcomes in adults due to the increased fusion of the mid-palate suture prior to puberty. However, Drs Christian Guilleminault, Stanley Liu, and Audrey Yoon at Stanford Medical Centre developed a protocol that achieves maximal bony expansion and nasal floor remodelling for adults with a narrow, high-arch palate called Distraction Osteogenesis Maxillary Expansion (DOME). The idea is to transform a gothic-shaped arch into a more dome-shaped form to improve the nasal airway. This will also allow more space for the tongue to fit and for tongue-to-palate contact to be restored.

DOME uses mini-implants placed in the bone near the mid-palate suture. These support an expansion device that delivers the expansion force more directly across the suture, ensuring it can be opened reliably.

A couple of relatively simple surgical cuts are made to separate the hard palate from the rest of the upper jaw or maxilla (refer to image) and the mid-palate suture is slightly wedged open at the front aspect. This minimises the transmission of large expansion forces throughout the upper facial and cranial structures. This surgery can be done extra-orally or with a modified and minimal approach through the nose.

These cuts make it easier for the palate bones to move with less resistance from the rest of the facial bones, as they do in childhood. Distraction osteogenesis can be achieved, and the need for a more invasive surgical procedure that was previously thought necessary can be eliminated.

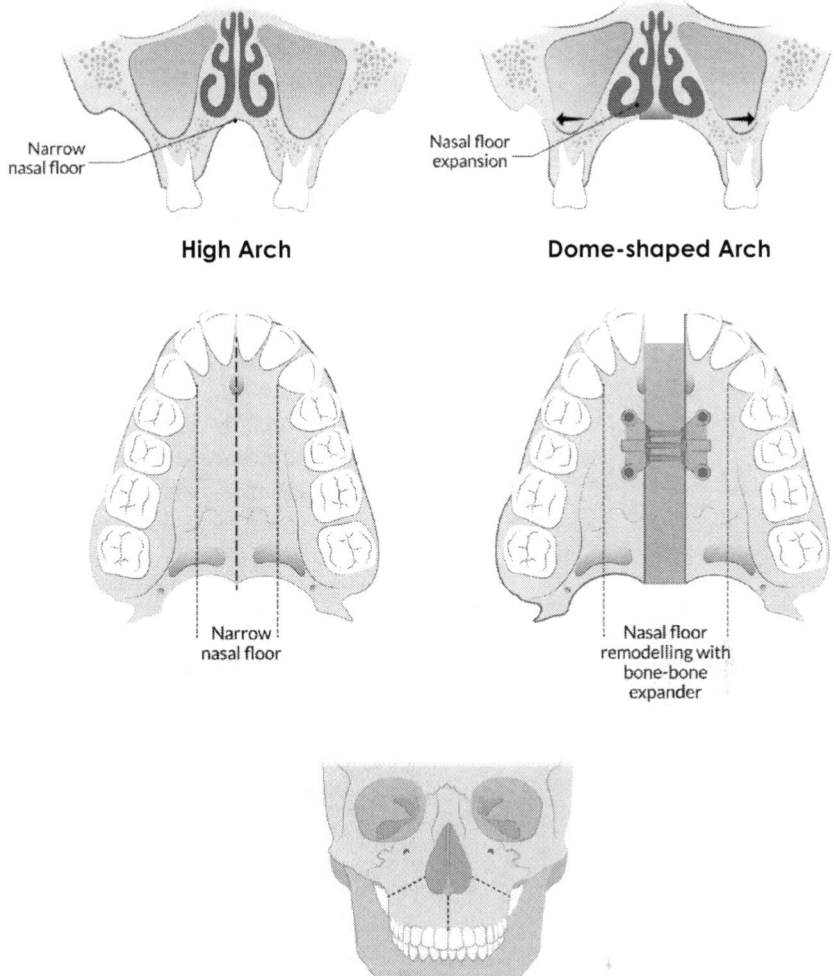

In January 2020, the results of a study of 75 patients who received this targeted anatomic intervention for adults with high, narrow palates were published in Sleep Medicine.[26] It was demonstrated DOME significantly reduces nasal congestion in patients with high-arch palates, significantly alleviates OSA, reduces daytime sleepiness, and increases time in REM sleep, which is very important for memory consolidation.

The team has reported one of the ways DOME is effective at reducing OSA is by decreasing nasal resistance and allowing smoother airflow, reducing upper airway collapsibility.[27] It also makes more space for the tongue to fit while restoring normal tongue-to-palate contact.

While there are various methods involving mini, implant-supported (also called bone borne) expanders available, so far DOME has the most data supporting its effectiveness and predictability in maximising nasal floor remodelling, reducing nasal congestion, and alleviating OSA, and the approach is continually evolving.

The experience of Dr Liu and other researchers at Stanford Medical Centre has shown it is also key to improving the effectiveness and stability of results of other OSA surgeries including nasal, soft palate, hypoglossal nerve stimulation, and the double jaw advancement surgery. Recent research has demonstrated that DOME is effective at reducing persistent nasal obstruction in patients with failed nasal septum surgery.[28] Another study by ENT surgeon Dr Eric Thuler included patients with failed soft palate and MMA surgeries.[29] Examination of their sites of airway collapse with the use of a video endoscope in the airway whilst under light sedation to mimic natural sleep found their OSA was associated with a narrow palate and tongue base obstruction. Again, we must not overlook the importance of having good palate structure, to improve predictability of results whenever other interventions are offered.

Case Study: 25-year-old year old male patient with a diagnosis of mild OSA

Kevin was a 25-year-old male patient who was diagnosed with mild OSA (AHI=10). He had severe nasal obstruction and excessive daytime sleepiness. He had been trialling multiple masks for CPAP and using a full-face mask but was not finding this option best for him. His provisional treatment plan included DOME as a Stage 1 surgery to address his narrow high arched palate. MMA surgery was proposed as a later Stage 2 surgery to address his recessed lower jaw.

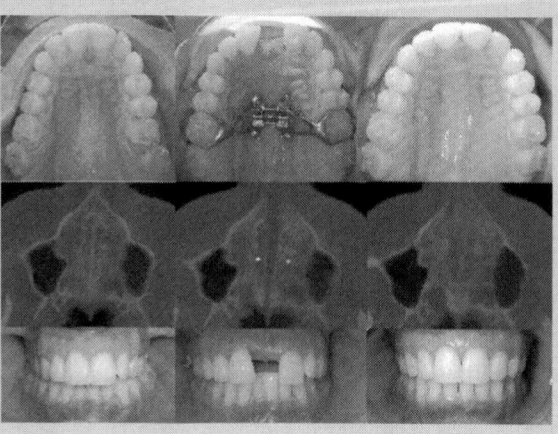

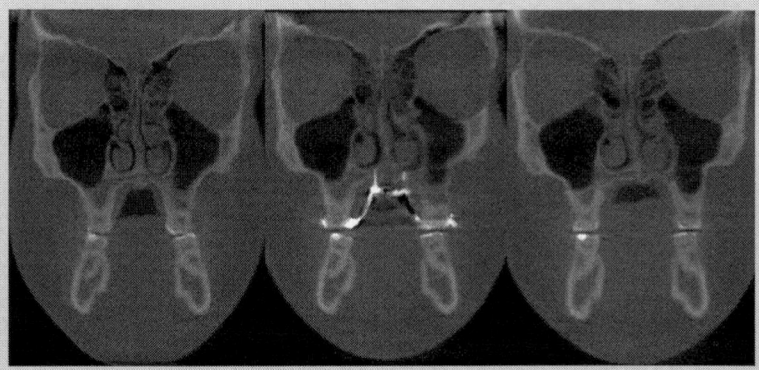

Photos shared and used with permission by Dr Audrey Yoon

These images represent pre-treatment, one-month of expansion in conjunction with surgery, and post-orthodontic treatment to close the space and correct the bite. They demonstrate remodelling and expansion of the nasal floor, improved tongue space, and improved tongue posture.

Following Kevin's palate expansion:

- OSA decreased from an AHI of 10 to 5.
- Epworth Sleepiness Scale (ESS) scores went from 18/24 (severe excessive daytime sleepiness) to 2/24 (normal).
- Nasal Obstruction Symptom Evaluation (NOSE) scores – which measure the severity of nasal congestion – went from 18/20 (extreme nasal congestion) to 0/20 (normal).

Since Kevin had such a significant improvement in breathing and symptoms, he was able to function more effectively throughout the day, and subsequently his Stage 2 MMA surgery was cancelled.

The high-arch palate is a common finding in many patients that present to me with a diagnosis of OSA. One of the big issues in helping patients access this treatment option is the lack of integration between specialties, something that we need more of.

At present, most orthodontic postgraduate programs in Australia do not offer extensive experience in the use of mini implants for palate expansion. There is also a greater need for the dental profession to recognise the functional benefits of palate expansion on nasal breathing and restoring tongue space, even when people have straight teeth.

However, the integration between specialities is starting to occur more with growing research, and training is being introduced in more orthodontic programs for example in the U.S.

Upper airway stimulation

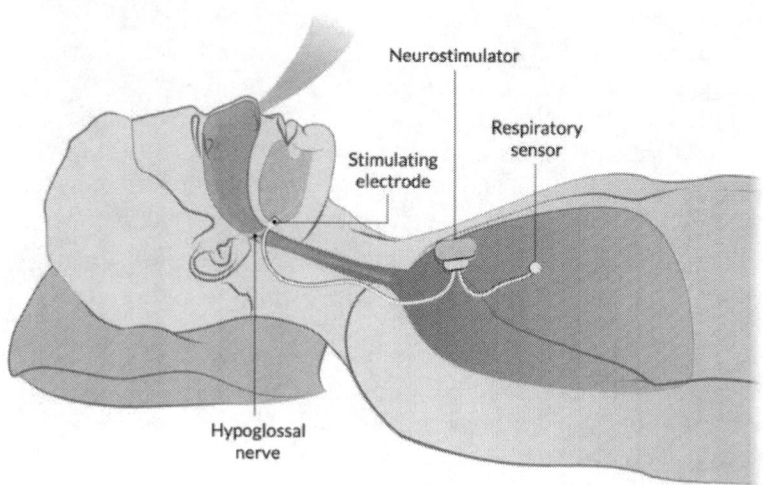

Upper Airway Stimulation, also called Hypoglossal Nerve Stimulation, is another highly effective treatment for moderate-to-severe OSA that is currently undergoing clinical trials for use in Australia.

The target of this treatment is to address poor muscle tone of the genioglossus muscle, which forms the bulk of the tongue. When this muscle contracts, it stabilises and enlarges the airway. It is the most important upper airway dilator muscle. When it relaxes, especially during sleep, the throat is particularly vulnerable to collapse.

Upper Airway Stimulation can be considered a 'pacemaker for the tongue.' It involves placing a sensor in the chest to detect breathing that is then synced to an electrical pulse generator implanted beneath the skin of the neck. This sends a signal to the hypoglossal nerve, the motor nerve of the tongue, to contract or increase tone of the tongue and prevent obstruction.

This may be a beneficial treatment for some patients who can't tolerate frontline options like CPAP or dental devices or don't want to have more invasive surgeries. It works best when the mouth is closed and there is enough room for the tongue. Combining it with skeletal surgeries like MMA and DOME can increase the overall effectiveness and reduce the voltage of stimulation required.

• • •

Stanford Sleep Surgeon Dr Stanley Liu performs and trains other surgeons to offer the full scope of sleep surgery including ENT and jaw surgeries (including MMA and DOME), and upper airway stimulation. He is also responsible for publishing recent updates to the 30-year-old Stanford Sleep Surgery Protocol that helps guide surgeons in selecting the most targeted and personalised surgeries for each individual. This makes him one of the most qualified people to discuss integrative team management of airway problems.

He suggests that no matter what the surgery to restore airway structure, the goal should be to re-educate and restore normal function through myofunctional therapy for lasting results. This means ensuring nasal breathing and good tone of the tongue and other muscles that keep the throat open. His observation is that palate expansion plays a central role in restoring this.

Despite what is possible to achieve these days in growing adults, the need for more invasive surgeries does involve risks. Our best opportunity is still to ensure optimal function and structural development from birth. This helps to set up the best trajectory of brain development, learning, and health from the earliest years of life while minimising the chances of debilitating consequences into adulthood.

12

THE FUTURE

As much as we want to treasure the earliest years of our child's life, it's important to remember that they will inevitably grow into adults, and we want to set them up as best as we can for the road ahead so they can be happy and healthy. Many of us can identify our own health status and experiences from the information throughout this book and recognise that we don't want our child to walk down the same path. The more proactive we can be, the better their future.

Much too often, constricted airways remain a hidden issue. By now, you should recognise that when air does not pass smoothly through the nose and down the throat during the day, we adopt compensations such as open mouth breathing, lowered tongue posture, forward head posture, and over breathing (fast and shallow breaths) to maintain airflow. No matter how much we compensate throughout our waking hours, narrow airways and breathing dysfunction will ultimately play out after we go to bed.

During sleep, when the muscles are relaxed, may be when problems stand out for the first time. Sleep disturbed breathing involves narrow airway structure and increased resistance to normal passage of air and leads to increased collapsibility of the throat during sleep. There is mounting research linking these breathing difficulties with many health risks including high blood pressure, heart disease, diabetes, obesity, depression, cancers, erectile dysfunction and more.

> We want children to be still, peaceful, and breathing quietly through their nose while they sleep so they can enter the deep, restorative phases. These characteristics paint the ideal picture of what we hope to achieve through the airway health movement.

The future of managing the burden of chronic diseases involves doing so through prevention. With the recognition of airway health, this includes paying attention to nasal breathing, mouth function, and jaw development in the earliest years of childhood.

I have now been involved in the team approach to managing adult OSA for over a decade. The way it affects each individual varies widely. The most despairing patients are those who have struggled all their life with hidden problems. It is not uncommon for me to meet those who report brain fog, not being able to access their full mental capacity, constantly feeling tired and unable to function properly at work, having no energy for their families, feeling depressed, and generally not enjoying life. As I listen to their histories, I see how many red flags and opportunities to intervene were missed early in life.

Often, these patients were children who had hidden allergies, mouth breathing, breastfeeding problems, difficulties concentrating at school, bedwetting, or crooked teeth. These are all indicators that a child could be at risk of developing problems down the road.

Kelly, a 35-year-old patient of mine, presented with worsening snoring to the point that she had to move into a separate room from her bed partner. She snored her whole life, even as a child. She couldn't breathe through her nose. She also had chronic neck pain and headaches. Kelly was chronically tired and in a constant state of brain fog, anxiety, and depression. She shared with me that she was physically, mentally, and emotionally struggling.

When she was younger, she had overcrowded teeth which were addressed with extractions and braces. However, her mouth was too small for her tongue to fit. Nobody addressed the actual issue of poor jaw development. They were just focused on straightening her teeth.

Delving even further into her history, as a baby, she had an undiagnosed tongue tie. Her mum couldn't breastfeed her because of painful latching. Kelly also had troubles with allergies her entire life. She had her adenoids and tonsils taken out as a child but continued to breathe through her mouth. She also had speech therapy for several years but didn't make much progress. Her first diagnosis of obstructive sleep apnoea was in her teenage years, but it was never addressed. Kelly was told to go on stimulant medications to improve daytime symptoms.

Kelly showed many clear warning signs of compromised airway health from the time she was a baby. If her parents and the healthcare professionals around her were more knowledgeable about the structure and function of good airway health, she could have been saved from years of downward spiraling conditions.

Our optimal health span begins in childhood, so it's crucial to pay more attention to airway health in our earliest years of life. We must acknowledge the problems and actively work toward a solution that will allow children to breathe, sleep and learn to their full potential so they don't turn into adults with persistent struggles.

My goal is to make airway health such a powerful movement that everyone becomes more aware and knowledgeable about it.

In today's age, people are quite effective at managing symptoms of poor airway health with drugs all the way through life. I believe that parents don't want to have their children on medications. It's not something built into their initial parenting plans, but as symptoms and diagnoses arise within a child, many parents put their trust in modern medicine recommendations by their healthcare providers. However, medicines are mere band-aids on the actual root problem. For example, the diagnosis of childhood ADHD is based on symptoms and observations in a clinical interview, which is subjective. These children may then be medicated with powerful stimulant medications with potentially serious side effects without anyone asking about their sleep.

Whilst healthcare focuses on researching new medications and surgeries, little attention is paid to properly functioning airways being a major pillar of health, and not much thought is given to the opportunity to prevent the development of even the earliest stage issues.

Airway health is focused on addressing the root cause of problems through a holistic view and integrative approach individualized to each patient's precise risk factors.

Here's an overview of traditional medicine and dentistry-focused vs. airway-focused approaches to care:

Traditional

- Treats symptoms of ADHD, anxiety, depression, high blood pressure, gastro-oesophageal reflux – with medication, and without any consideration of sleep and breathing history.
- Focused on OSA as an end point disease or a number, meaning breathing disturbance must be severe enough to meet criteria for diagnosis. A lot of people have undiagnosed breathing difficulties and get labelled or medicated unnecessarily.
- Treatment of OSA often involves band-aid solutions which splint the airway open during sleep, such as CPAP and dental devices, but these don't help re-establish better airway structure and function or nasal breathing during the day.

- Crooked teeth are addressed by watchful waiting and straightening with braces, sometimes including extractions without addressing poor jaw development.
- Adenoids and tonsils are removed in children without anybody asking why they got so large in the first place.
- Healthcare is compartmentalized, meaning an adult may go to a psychologist and be put on antidepressants, see a specialist for headaches, high blood pressure, and so on. No one is seeing their full health picture.
- Speech concerns are addressed by a speech pathologist, and children may also have a psychologist, a dentist to fix mouth decay, and a bedwetting alarm, or they may require special education. All these issues stem from airway dysfunction and solely treating them avoids addressing the core problem.
- Myofunctional disorders such as infant latching, picky eating, lisping, etc. are all treated individually – no dots are connected between sucking, swallowing, speech and breathing and there is no recognition these are early markers of airway problems.

Airway health

- Not so focused on numbers and arbitrary cut-offs to define disease – it's about moving towards optimal health and wellness.
- Recognises that healthy nasal breathing is a key pillar of good health and wellness, and is integral for good sleep, mood, learning and much more. It is worthy of as much attention as healthy diets and exercise.
- Recognises mouth breathing, snoring and audible breathing, crooked teeth, and myofunctional disorders as warning signs of problems ahead.
- Addresses poor jaw development early when children are growing most rapidly. At the same time, the underlying poor muscle patterns that have contributed to the problem are addressed.
- Teeth are not extracted for the sole purpose of alleviating dental crowding.
- Views enlarged adenoids and tonsils as a symptom, rather than their removal being a cure. Root causes are addressed following ENT surgery to minimise the recurrence of symptoms and need for repeated surgeries.
- Child health professionals and educators are fully informed about the importance of good airway and sleep health. Every child is screened for airway and breathing problems when they have speech and feeding issues or before they are labelled with behavioural or learning problems.

- All infants are screened for tongue-tie at birth and the mechanical benefits of breastfeeding are promoted. All health care professionals involved in the care of infants understand the big picture: that we need the tongue to work well for other functions, and good jaw and airway development. We look beyond the goal of "no pain, good weight gain" and look beyond nipple shields, or bottle feeding and formula as solutions when there are problems, to see if oral function can be optimised.

- Dental professionals act as quarterbacks of the airway. They help screen for hidden airway problems and poor airway development, and co-ordinate integrative team care to address risk factors and problems. Mouth breathing is recognised as a risk factor when there is decay, inflamed gums, orthodontic problems or poor jaw development, teeth wear related to teeth grinding or reflux disease, or bad breath.

- Less focus on managing chronic health disease and research on new medications, and more focus on early intervention, including pre-maternal influences. For example, if we know premature babies have an increased risk of oral dysfunction and poor jaw development, the airway health approach looks at how we can prevent pre-term births and considers making sure mothers have good airway health, because maternal OSA is linked to increased risk of eclampsia, intra-uterine growth restriction, and pre-term births. Or if we know allergies contribute to the development of nasal congestion and mouth breathing, it considers what mothers do during pregnancy or delivery to alter that or influence their microbiome.

- Offers patients with sleep-disturbed breathing a choice to re-establish normal airway structure and function rather than relying on band-aid solutions. In adults it's recognizing that this may involve jaw surgery, such as adult palate expansion or double jaw advancement. Patients can opt for a path towards greater wellness instead of just addressing night-time problems.

- Surgery or orthodontic treatment to address jaw deficiency is combined with re-education to restore nasal breathing, tongue tone, and other muscle patterns.

The future of sleep medicine for obstructive breathing is precision and personalized management. This means rather than relying on generalized treatments such as removal of enlarged adenoids and tonsils, CPAP, and MAD, patients are offered more tailored combinations of options that precisely target their individual risk factors and suit their preferences.

But an even loftier goal is to promote airway health – and to recognise the progression of sleep breathing problems begins when mouth breathing starts, and long before the oxygen deprivation kicks in. It is through being educated as parents and having more awareness of our own health that we notice airway restriction as soon as signs appear. We need to promote nasal breathing in our children in the earliest years of life, when so many of the body's organs and systems – as well as the jaw and airway – are developing rapidly. We have a lot of influence over a child's trajectory of airway and breathing if we know what to look for.

In children, screening through history and clinical examination may identify signs and symptoms of deficient growth and development, or other risk factors that may lead to airway issues. Right now, dental professionals are the so-called gatekeepers of the airway. We see patients more regularly and spend more time with them than their pediatrician or GP. When dentists are properly trained, they can identify deficient jaw growth, clues in the mouth, and instigate necessary referrals. An airway-focused dental practice will be the best place to start to set your child on the right health track if any symptoms have been presented.

This book's goal isn't to make you feel guilty if you haven't taken proper action for a symptom your child has expressed. What I want to do is empower you to help lead the charge of a paradigm shift in how we approach these symptoms and encourage other parents in the process. It is common for us to be told children will grow out of problems, but they most often grow around and into new ones. That's why we need to move from band aid solutions to address root causes. When it comes to the grand scheme of life, it takes a relatively short amount of time to address concerns and identify and treat the root cause to restore normal function and development. By being an aware, proactive advocate for your child's airway health, you are saving hours, weeks, months, or years of tears, frustration, and sleepless nights – but most of all, you're avoiding the aftermath of compounding problems, which can be detrimental to you and your child's long-term mental, emotional, and physical health. As parents, we recognise the yearning to protect our children in every way we can.

Airway health, optimal breathing, and restorative sleep matter, and I hope you now have the knowledge to represent a movement that will create generational change in health and our expectations of care for not only our children, but future lifelines.

ACKNOWLEDGMENTS

There are many people who have inspired and supported me throughout the long journey of finalising this book, and who I would like to shout my thanks to!

Firstly, I'd like to acknowledge the late sleep medicine and obstructive sleep apnoea pioneer Dr Christian Guilleminault, also affectionately known as CG. He inspired many of us across the globe with his discoveries, passion, and imagination of a future where we could prevent obstructive sleep apnoea, by taking action early in childhood. It was his work that prompted me to learn more about interceptive orthodontics, and when I shared this with him in 2014, his comment "if you're doing palate expansion, you're too late," ignited my curiosity and search for more answers to discover more about root causes of poor jaw development, myofunctional therapy and tongue tie – shaping everything I do in practice today. His pleas to "save the children," stirred me to keep spreading the message, and this book is ultimately one of many wide-reaching ripples from the original ideas he cast.

The following key thought leaders were my original influences in early intervention - Drs Jeff Rouse, Derek Mahony, Barry Raphael, Bill Hang, German Ramirez, Kevin Boyd, and Larry Kotlow. Thank you for your great influence, and all the work you have done paving the way for all of us and the better health and wellness of countless children around the world!

My more recent inspirations Drs Audrey Yoon, Stanley Liu and Soroush Zaghi who I met in Chicago March 2017 – I'm a massive fan of all your fantastic work and research contributions and thank you for all you do to validate CG's ideas, advance greater integrative care in sleep medicine and promote airway health. I'm grateful to count you superstars as friends! Thank you, Audrey, for the extra support and contribution in the way of case studies.

Thank you to the many other countless friends and colleagues who I have enjoyed travel, discussions and learning from and together with. It's exciting times to share this journey and see the growing momentum behind a collaborative care for airway health all around the world!

A special thank you to the AAPMD Endeavour crew who I have met online with every week for the past two years to brainstorm how to further professional and public awareness so that more children can access early treatment to optimise airway health. These conversations have greatly influenced the direction of the book.

I'm grateful to book coach Lauren Eckhart from Burning Soul Press for believing in the importance of this book, and for ensuring the best structure moving forward. Your constant enthusiasm, encouragement, support, and feedback to make each version of the manuscript more parent-centric breathed new life and inspiration into this project. Thank you to my dental and Endeavour colleague Dr Susan Maples for introducing me to you!

To Allison, Claire, and Lauren, at Burning Soul Press. Thank you, Allison, for your thorough proofing of the manuscript. Whilst the book formatting process was one of the most challenging experiences I have endured, I am grateful that you all listened, took ownership, and took over the job, working around the clock to make things right fast. It says a lot about your care, character, and what your business stands for. It has meant a lot to me to work with a team that I could rely upon to care about the details as much as I did, especially when things got tough. A special congrats to Allison on your can-do attitude and a surprisingly efficient and wonderful first-time job with book formatting, worth celebrating!

To my general accountability coach Darren Finkelstein. Thank you for your care and support through the challenges and struggles, and for keeping me focused to see this through to the end.

Thank you to my dear friend Aisha Timol, inspirational colleague Dr Steve Cartensen, and passionate parent advocate and supporter Hannah How for taking the time to review an earlier manuscript, and providing much needed feedback, care, support and offers to help along the way!

Thank you to Dorothy Nelson for your invaluable check ins, support and encouragement, and your time and efforts, reviewing and sharing feedback towards the completion of this project. I deeply value your care and friendship and forget that we have not even met in person. I look forward to doing so soon!

A shout out of thanks to our practice manager Karli for the awesome job she does at work and with our team. I feel I can achieve anything with your constant support and help to take care of all the details! I'm lucky to have such an amazing cheerleader. Thank you for all the "adult stickers!"

Thank you also to the rest of our Sparkle team for their support and dedication to creating wonderful experiences for our patients and families! I couldn't do what I do and continually learn through so many patient journeys without them and their terrific engagement with children!

I've been extremely lucky to have had many opportunities to have travelled far and wide over the years to learn from the very best leaders in the field who have shaped my thinking. The knowledge I've acquired, and connections made, could not have happened without the support of my parents and James and Lena Lim, and in-laws Peter and Christobelle Devellerez, especially when our girls were much younger. Thank you for all you do, especially ensuring that they have never been in doubt of how loved, cared for and special they are.

And lastly to the loves of my life -

Our incredible daughters Jessica and Chloe - a lot of what I was driven to learn was because I wanted to help them avoid growing into the problems I'd seen in my adult patients. They were my guinea pigs for lots of new things I learned along the way, and I thank them for putting up with my constant talk of tongues and breathing, and requests to look in their mouths! I am proud of them in every imaginable way.

And Alex - my husband, best friend, and partner in crime. My interest in breathing and sleep all began with his snoring - so you could say that was one of his biggest gifts to me! Thank you for all your patience, and support whilst I've travelled, learned, and obsessed about spreading more awareness and knowledge on these topics through organising conferences, preparing talks, and the roller coaster ride of writing this book!

I love my work and making a difference to help more people sleep and breathe easier fulfils me every day. But it is your pride and the shared excitement as this chapter ends and being able to enjoy this beautiful family and life, we have created together that completes me!

REFERENCES

Chapter 1: Sleep and Breathing

1. The Urban Child Institute, "Baby's Brain Begins Now: Conception to Age 3." Accessed 10 July 2022, http://www.urbanchildinstitute.org/why-0-3/baby-and-brain
2. Thomas, S., Patel, S., Gummalla, P., Tablizo, M. A., & Kier, C. (2022). You Cannot Hit Snooze on OSA: Sequelae of Pediatric Obstructive Sleep Apnea. *Children (Basel, Switzerland), 9*(2), 261. https://doi.org/10.3390/children9020261
3. Zaffanello, M., Piacentini, G., & La Grutta, S. (2020). The cardiovascular risk in paediatrics: the paradigm of the obstructive sleep apnoea syndrome. *Blood transfusion = Trasfusione del sangue, 18*(3), 217–225. https://doi.org/10.2450/2020.0283-19
4. Trosman, I., & Trosman, S. J. (2017). Cognitive and Behavioral Consequences of Sleep Disordered Breathing in Children. *Medical sciences (Basel, Switzerland), 5*(4), 30. https://doi.org/10.3390/medsci5040030
5. Hunter, S. J., Gozal, D., Smith, D. L., Philby, M. F., Kaylegian, J., & Kheirandish-Gozal, L. (2016). Effect of Sleep-disordered Breathing Severity on Cognitive Performance Measures in a Large Community Cohort of Young School-aged Children. *American journal of respiratory and critical care medicine, 194*(6), 739–747. https://doi.org/10.1164/rccm.201510-2099OC
6. Smith, D. L., Gozal, D., Hunter, S. J., & Kheirandish-Gozal, L. (2017). Frequency of snoring, rather than apnea-hypopnea index, predicts both cognitive and behavioral problems in young children. *Sleep medicine, 34*, 170–178. https://doi.org/10.1016/j.sleep.2017.02.028
7. Sedky, K., Bennett, D. S., & Carvalho, K. S. (2014). Attention deficit hyperactivity disorder and sleep disordered breathing in pediatric populations: a meta-analysis. *Sleep medicine reviews, 18*(4), 349–356. https://doi.org/10.1016/j.smrv.2013.12.003
8. Urbano, G. L., Tablizo, B. J., Moufarrej, Y., Tablizo, M. A., Chen, M. L., & Witmans, M. (2021). The Link between Pediatric Obstructive Sleep Apnea (OSA) and Attention Deficit Hyperactivity Disorder (ADHD). *Children (Basel, Switzerland), 8*(9), 824. https://doi.org/10.3390/children8090824
9. Bonuck, K., Freeman, K., Chervin, R. D., & Xu, L. (2012). Sleep-disordered breathing in a population-based cohort: behavioral outcomes at 4 and 7 years. *Pediatrics, 129*(4), e857–e865. https://doi.org/10.1542/peds.2011-1402
10. Marcus, C. L., Brooks, L. J., Draper, K. A., Gozal, D., Halbower, A. C., Jones, J., Schechter, M. S., Ward, S. D., Sheldon, S. H., Shiffman, R. N., Lehmann, C.,

Spruyt, K., & American Academy of Pediatrics (2012). Diagnosis and management of childhood obstructive sleep apnea syndrome. *Pediatrics*, *130*(3), e714–e755. https://doi.org/10.1542/peds.2012-1672

11. Isaiah, A., Ernst, T., Cloak, C.C. *et al.* Associations between frontal lobe structure, parent-reported obstructive sleep disordered breathing and childhood behavior in the ABCD dataset. *Nat Commun* **12**, 2205 (2021). https://doi.org/10.1038/s41467-021-22534-0

12. Menzies, B., Teng, A., Burns, M., & Lah, S. (2022). Neurocognitive outcomes of children with sleep disordered breathing: A systematic review with meta-analysis. *Sleep medicine reviews*, *63*, 101629. https://doi.org/10.1016/j.smrv.2022.101629

13. Gozal D. (1998). Sleep-disordered breathing and school performance in children. *Pediatrics*, *102*(3 Pt 1), 616–620. https://doi.org/10.1542/peds.102.3.616

14. Gozal, D., & Pope, D. W., Jr (2001). Snoring during early childhood and academic performance at ages thirteen to fourteen years. *Pediatrics*, *107*(6), 1394–1399. https://doi.org/10.1542/peds.107.6.1394

15. Science Daily, "Untreated sleep apnea in children can harm brain cells tied to cognition and mood." March 17, 2017, https://www.sciencedaily.com/releases/2017/03/170317082507.htm

16. Ask an Orthodontist, with Dr Derek Mahony. 2022. *Putting Sleep Problems to Bed, with Professor David Gozal*. [online] Available at: <https://podcasts.apple.com/ca/podcast/putting-sleep-problems-to-bed-with-professor-david-gozal/id1584676501?i=1000543447671> [Accessed 10 July 2022].

17. Bhattacharjee, R., Kheirandish-Gozal, L., Spruyt, K., Mitchell, R. B., Promchiarak, J., Simakajornboon, N., Kaditis, A. G., Splaingard, D., Splaingard, M., Brooks, L. J., Marcus, C. L., Sin, S., Arens, R., Verhulst, S. L., & Gozal, D. (2010). Adenotonsillectomy outcomes in treatment of obstructive sleep apnea in children: a multicenter retrospective study. *American journal of respiratory and critical care medicine*, *182*(5), 676–683. https://doi.org/10.1164/rccm.200912-1930OC

18. Tasker, C., Crosby, J. H., & Stradling, J. R. (2002). Evidence for persistence of upper airway narrowing during sleep, 12 years after adenotonsillectomy. *Archives of disease in childhood*, *86*(1), 34–37. https://doi.org/10.1136/adc.86.1.34

19. Guilleminault, C., Huang, Y. S., Quo, S., Monteyrol, P. J., & Lin, C. H. (2013). Teenage sleep-disordered breathing: recurrence of syndrome. *Sleep medicine*, *14*(1), 37–44. https://doi.org/10.1016/j.sleep.2012.08.010

Chapter 2: Airway Health

1. Edwards, C., Mukherjee, S., Simpson, L., Palmer, L. J., Almeida, O. P., & Hillman, D. R. (2015). Depressive Symptoms before and after Treatment of Obstructive Sleep Apnea in Men and Women. *Journal of clinical sleep medicine*

: *JCSM : official publication of the American Academy of Sleep Medicine*, *11*(9), 1029–1038. https://doi.org/10.5664/jcsm.5020

2. Oscullo, G., Torres, G., Campos-Rodriguez, F., Posadas, T., Reina-González, A., Sapiña-Beltrán, E., Barbé, F., & Martinez-Garcia, M. A. (2019). Resistant/Refractory Hypertension and Sleep Apnoea: Current Knowledge and Future Challenges. *Journal of clinical medicine*, *8*(11), 1872. https://doi.org/10.3390/jcm8111872

3. Guilleminault, C., Huang, Y. S., Chin, W. C., & Okorie, C. (2019). The nocturnal-polysomnogram and "non-hypoxic sleep-disordered-breathing" in children. *Sleep medicine*, *60*, 31–44. https://doi.org/10.1016/j.sleep.2018.11.001

4. Bai, J., He, B., Wang, N., Chen, Y., Liu, J., Wang, H., & Liu, D. (2021). Snoring Is Associated With Increased Risk of Stroke: A Cumulative Meta-Analysis. *Frontiers in neurology*, *12*, 574649. https://doi.org/10.3389/fneur.2021.574649

5. Liao, Felix. *Six-foot tiger, three-foot cage*. Carlsbad: Crescendo Publishing, 2017

6. Medium. "Our Skulls Are Out-Evolving Us." September 19, 2019, https://onezero.medium.com/our-skulls-are-out-evolving-us-and-that-could-mean-a-public-health-crisis-f950faed696d

7. Boyd, Kevin. (2012). Darwinian Dentistry Part 2: early childhood nutrition, dentofacial development and chronic disease. *Journal of the American Orthodontic Society*. 12. 28-32.

8. Kahn, S., Ehrlich, P., Feldman, M., Sapolsky, R., & Wong, S. (2020). The Jaw Epidemic: Recognition, Origins, Cures, and Prevention. *Bioscience*, *70*(9), 759–771. https://doi.org/10.1093/biosci/biaa073

9. Kahn, S. and Ehrlich, *Jaws: The Story of a Hidden Epidemic*. Stanford University Press, 2018

10. Guilleminault, C., & Akhtar, F. (2015). Pediatric sleep-disordered breathing: New evidence on its development. *Sleep medicine reviews*, *24*, 46–56. https://doi.org/10.1016/j.smrv.2014.11.008

11. Guilleminault, C., & Huang, Y. S. (2018). From oral facial dysfunction to dysmorphism and the onset of pediatric OSA. *Sleep medicine reviews*, *40*, 203–214. https://doi.org/10.1016/j.smrv.2017.06.008

12. Huang, Y. S., Hsu, J. F., Paiva, T., Chin, W. C., Chen, I. C., & Guilleminault, C. (2019). Sleep-disordered breathing, craniofacial development, and neurodevelopment in premature infants: a 2-year follow-up study. *Sleep medicine*, *60*, 20–25. https://doi.org/10.1016/j.sleep.2018.10.015

Chapter 3: Mouth Breathing

1. Abreu, R. R., Rocha, R. L., Lamounier, J. A., & Guerra, A. F. (2008). Prevalence of mouth breathing among children. *Jornal de pediatria*, *84*(5), 467–470. https://doi.org/10.2223/JPED.1806

2. Caitlyn, George. Shut your mouth and save your life. Trubner, 1882

3. Nestor, James. *Breath: The New Science of A Lost Art*. London, UK: Penguin, 2020

4. Kukwa, W., Guilleminault, C., Tomaszewska, M., Kukwa, A., Krzeski, A., & Migacz, E. (2018). Prevalence of upper respiratory tract infections in habitually snoring and mouth breathing children. *International journal of pediatric otorhinolaryngology, 107*, 37–41. https://doi.org/10.1016/j.ijporl.2018.01.022

5. Izuhara, Y., Matsumoto, H., Nagasaki, T., Kanemitsu, Y., Murase, K., Ito, I., Oguma, T., Muro, S., Asai, K., Tabara, Y., Takahashi, K., Bessho, K., Sekine, A., Kosugi, S., Yamada, R., Nakayama, T., Matsuda, F., Niimi, A., Chin, K., Mishima, M., ... Nagahama Study Group (2016). Mouth breathing, another risk factor for asthma: the Nagahama Study. *Allergy, 71*(7), 1031–1036. https://doi.org/10.1111/all.12885

6. Bueno, D., Grechi, T. H., Trawitzki, L. V., Anselmo-Lima, W. T., Felício, C. M., & Valera, F. C. (2015). Muscular and functional changes following adenotonsillectomy in children. *International journal of pediatric otorhinolaryngology, 79*(4), 537–540. https://doi.org/10.1016/j.ijporl.2015.01.024

7. Valera, F. C., Trawitzki, L. V., & Anselmo-Lima, W. T. (2006). Myofunctional evaluation after surgery for tonsils hypertrophy and its correlation to breathing pattern: a 2-year-follow up. *International journal of pediatric otorhinolaryngology, 70*(2), 221–225. https://doi.org/10.1016/j.ijporl.2005.06.005

8. Jefferson Y. (2010). Mouth breathing: adverse effects on facial growth, health, academics, and behavior. *General dentistry, 58*(1), 18–80.

9. Sullivan, S. S., & Guilleminault, C. (2017). Can we avoid development of a narrow upper airway and secondary abnormal breathing during sleep?. *The Lancet. Respiratory medicine, 5*(11), 843–844. https://doi.org/10.1016/S2213-2600(17)30351-X

10. Fitzpatrick, M. F., McLean, H., Urton, A. M., Tan, A., O'Donnell, D., & Driver, H. S. (2003). Effect of nasal or oral breathing route on upper airway resistance during sleep. *The European respiratory journal, 22*(5), 827–832. https://doi.org/10.1183/09031936.03.00047903

11. Catalano PJ, Walker J. ADD & ADHD in Children: The Answer is Right in Their Nose. Am J Otolaryngol Head Neck Surg. 2018; 1(5): 1025.

12. Kalaskar, R., Bhaje, P., Kalaskar, A., & Faye, A. (2021). Sleep Difficulties and Symptoms of Attention-deficit Hyperactivity Disorder in Children with Mouth Breathing. *International journal of clinical pediatric dentistry, 14*(5), 604–609. https://doi.org/10.5005/jp-journals-10005-1987

13. Bonuck, K., Freeman, K., Chervin, R. D., & Xu, L. (2012). Sleep-disordered breathing in a population-based cohort: behavioral outcomes at 4 and 7 years. *Pediatrics, 129*(4), e857–e865. https://doi.org/10.1542/peds.2011-1402

14. Bonuck, K., Rao, T., & Xu, L. (2012). Pediatric sleep disorders and special educational need at 8 years: a population-based cohort study. *Pediatrics, 130*(4), 634–642. https://doi.org/10.1542/peds.2012-0392

15. Lima, A., Albuquerque, R. C., Cunha, D., Lima, C., Lima, S., & Silva, H. (2021). Relation of sensory processing and stomatognical system of oral respiratory children. Relação do processamento sensorial e sistema estomatognático de crianças respiradoras orais. *CoDAS, 34*(2), e20200251. https://doi.org/10.1590/2317-1782/20212020251

16. Kaido, T., Hirabayashi, H., Murase, N., Sasaki, R., Shimokawara, T., Nagata, K., Bando, C., & Aono, Y. (2020). Deep slow nasal respiration with tight lip closure for immediate attenuation of severe tics. *Journal of clinical neuroscience : official journal of the Neurosurgical Society of Australasia*, *77*, 67–74. https://doi.org/10.1016/j.jocn.2020.05.037

17. Neiva, P. D., Kirkwood, R. N., Mendes, P. L., Zabjek, K., Becker, H. G., & Mathur, S. (2018). Postural disorders in mouth breathing children: a systematic review. *Brazilian journal of physical therapy*, *22*(1), 7–19. https://doi.org/10.1016/j.bjpt.2017.06.011

18. Abreu, R. R., Rocha, R. L., Lamounier, J. A., & Guerra, A. F. (2008). Etiology, clinical manifestations and concurrent findings in mouth-breathing children. *Jornal de pediatria*, *84*(6), 529–535. https://doi.org/10.2223/JPED.1844

19. Soroush Zaghi, Cynthia Peterson, Shayan Shamtoob, Brigitte Fung, Daniel Kwok-keung Ng, Triin Jagomagi, Nicole Archambault, Bridget O'Connor, Kathy Winslow, Zahra Peeran, Miche' Lano, Janine Murdock, Sanda Valcu-Pinkerton, Lenore Morrissey, Assessment of Nasal Breathing Using Lip Taping: A Simple and Effective Screening Tool, *International Journal of Otorhinolaryngology*. Volume 6, Issue 1, June 2020 , pp. 10-15. https://doi.org/10.11648/j.ijo.20200601.13

20. Torre, C., & Guilleminault, C. (2018). Establishment of nasal breathing should be the ultimate goal to secure adequate craniofacial and airway development in children. *Jornal de pediatria*, *94*(2), 101–103. https://doi.org/10.1016/j.jped.2017.08.002

21. Guilleminault C, Sullivan SS (2014) Towards Restoration of Continuous Nasal Breathing as the Ultimate Treatment Goal in Pediatric Obstructive Sleep Apnea. Enliven: Pediatr Neonatol Biol 1(1): 001.

Chapter 4: Infant Feeding and Sucking Habits

1. Geddes, D. T., Kent, J. C., Mitoulas, L. R., & Hartmann, P. E. (2008). Tongue movement and intra-oral vacuum in breastfeeding infants. *Early human development*, *84*(7), 471–477. https://doi.org/10.1016/j.earlhumdev.2007.12.008

2. Peres, K. G., Cascaes, A. M., Nascimento, G. G., & Victora, C. G. (2015). Effect of breastfeeding on malocclusions: a systematic review and meta-analysis. *Acta paediatrica (Oslo, Norway : 1992)*, *104*(467), 54–61. https://doi.org/10.1111/apa.13103

3. Thomaz, E., Alves, C., Gomes E Silva, L. F., Ribeiro de Almeida, C., Soares de Britto E Alves, M., Hilgert, J. B., & Wendland, E. M. (2018). Breastfeeding Versus Bottle Feeding on Malocclusion in Children: A Meta-Analysis Study. *Journal of human lactation : official journal of International Lactation Consultant Association*, *34*(4), 768–788. https://doi.org/10.1177/0890334418755689

4. Doğramacı, E. J., Rossi-Fedele, G., & Dreyer, C. W. (2017). Malocclusions in young children: Does breast-feeding really reduce the risk? A systematic review

and meta-analysis. *Journal of the American Dental Association (1939)*, *148*(8), 566–574.e6. https://doi.org/10.1016/j.adaj.2017.05.018

5. Peres, K. G., Cascaes, A. M., Peres, M. A., Demarco, F. F., Santos, I. S., Matijasevich, A., & Barros, A. J. (2015). Exclusive Breastfeeding and Risk of Dental Malocclusion. *Pediatrics*, *136*(1), e60–e67. https://doi.org/10.1542/peds.2014-3276

6. Neiva, F.C., Cattoni, D., Ramos, J., & Issler, H. (2003). [Early weaning: implications to oral motor development]. *Jornal de pediatria, 79 1*, 7-12 .

7. Pires, S. C., Giugliani, E. R., & Caramez da Silva, F. (2012). Influence of the duration of breastfeeding on quality of muscle function during mastication in preschoolers: a cohort study. *BMC public health*, *12*(1), 934. https://doi.org/10.1186/1471-2458-12-934

8. Storari, M., Yanez-Regonesi, F., Denotti, G., Paglia, L., & Viscuso, D. (2021). Breastfeeding and sleep-disordered breathing in children: systematic review and proposal of underlying interaction models. *European journal of paediatric dentistry*, *22*(4), 309–313. https://doi.org/10.23804/ejpd.2021.22.04.10

9. Vinha, P. P., & de Mello-Filho, F. V. (2017). Evidence of a Preventive Effect of Breastfeeding on Obstructive Sleep Apnea in Children and Adults. *Journal of human lactation : official journal of International Lactation Consultant Association*, *33*(2), 448–453. https://doi.org/10.1177/0890334416682006

10. Pitman, T. and Newman, J. *Dr. Jack Newman's guide to breastfeeding*. London: Pinter & Martin, 2019

11. Hauck, F. R., Omojokun, O. O., & Siadaty, M. S. (2005). Do pacifiers reduce the risk of sudden infant death syndrome? A meta-analysis. *Pediatrics*, *116*(5), e716–e723. https://doi.org/10.1542/peds.2004-2631

12. Levrini, L. The Effect of Pacifiers on Developmental Breathing Patterns. Presentation for Academy of Applied Myofunctional Sciences, Virtual Congress, August 2020

13. Zavala Abed, B., Oneto, S., Abreu, A. R., & Chediak, A. D. (2020). How might non nutritional sucking protect from sudden infant death syndrome. *Medical hypotheses*, *143*, 109868. https://doi.org/10.1016/j.mehy.2020.109868

14. Chen, X., Xia, B., & Ge, L. (2015). Effects of breast-feeding duration, bottle-feeding duration and non-nutritive sucking habits on the occlusal characteristics of primary dentition. *BMC pediatrics*, *15*, 46. https://doi.org/10.1186/s12887-015-0364-1

15. Doğramacı, E. J., & Rossi-Fedele, G. (2016). Establishing the association between nonnutritive sucking behavior and malocclusions: A systematic review and meta-analysis. *Journal of the American Dental Association (1939)*, *147*(12), 926–934.e6. https://doi.org/10.1016/j.adaj.2016.08.018

16. Schmid, K. M., Kugler, R., Nalabothu, P., Bosch, C., & Verna, C. (2018). The effect of pacifier sucking on orofacial structures: a systematic literature review. *Progress in orthodontics*, *19*(1), 8. https://doi.org/10.1186/s40510-018-0206-4

17. Bruderer, A. G., Danielson, D. K., Kandhadai, P., & Werker, J. F. (2015). Sensorimotor influences on speech perception in infancy. *Proceedings of the National Academy of Sciences of the United States of America*, *112*(44), 13531–13536. https://doi.org/10.1073/pnas.1508631112

18. Rychlowska, M., & Vanderwert, R. (2020). The Pacified Face: Early Embodiment Processes and the Use of Dummies. *Frontiers in psychology, 11*, 387. https://doi.org/10.3389/fpsyg.2020.00387
19. Nihi, V. S., Maciel, S. M., Jarrus, M. E., Nihi, F. M., Salles, C. L., Pascotto, R. C., & Fujimaki, M. (2015). Pacifier-sucking habit duration and frequency on occlusal and myofunctional alterations in preschool children. Brazilian oral research, 29, 1–7. https://doi.org/10.1590/1807-3107bor-2015.vol29.0013
20. Medeiros, R., Ximenes, M., Massignan, C., Flores-Mir, C., Vieira, R., Porporatti, A. L., & De Luca Canto, G. (2018). Malocclusion prevention through the usage of an orthodontic pacifier compared to a conventional pacifier: a systematic review. *European archives of paediatric dentistry : official journal of the European Academy of Paediatric Dentistry, 19*(5), 287–295. https://doi.org/10.1007/s40368-018-0359-3
21. Cook Country Record, "Judge allows class action to crawl ahead accusing maker of Nuk pacifiers of false advertising." November 23 2021, https://cookcountyrecord.com/stories/613245692-judge-allows-class-action-to-crawl-ahead-accusing-maker-of-nuk-pacifiers-of-false-advertising
22. Ferrante, A., & Ferrante, A. (2015). [Finger or thumb sucking. New interpretations and therapeutic implications]. *Minerva pediatrica, 67 4*, 285-97
23. Ferrante, A. The importance of myofunctional therapy for restoration of brain function. Presentation for the Academy of Applied Myofunctional Sciences Congress, Los Angeles, September 2015
24. Rapley, G. and Murkett, T., *Baby-led weaning.* London: Vermilion, 2008
25. New York Times, "Re-thinking food pouches." Accessed 10 July 2022. https://www.nytimes.com/2018/06/19/well/rethinking-baby-food-pouches.html
26. ABC News, "Are we raising 'generation suck' who drink food with no need for chewing." August 26, 2016 https://www.abc.net.au/news/rural/2016-08-26/generation-suck-could-damage-childrens-development/7787610

Chapter 5: Tongue-Ties

1. Bin-Nun, A., Kasirer, Y. M., & Mimouni, F. B. (2017). A Dramatic Increase in Tongue Tie-Related Articles: A 67 Years Systematic Review. *Breastfeeding medicine : the official journal of the Academy of Breastfeeding Medicine, 12*(7), 410–414. https://doi.org/10.1089/bfm.2017.0044
2. Ghaheri, B. A., Cole, M., Fausel, S. C., Chuop, M., & Mace, J. C. (2017). Breastfeeding improvement following tongue-tie and lip-tie release: A prospective cohort study. *The Laryngoscope, 127*(5), 1217–1223. https://doi.org/10.1002/lary.26306
3. Ghaheri, B. A., Cole, M., & Mace, J. C. (2018). Revision Lingual Frenotomy Improves Patient-Reported Breastfeeding Outcomes: A Prospective Cohort Study. *Journal of human lactation : official journal of International Lactation Consultant Association, 34*(3), 566–574. https://doi.org/10.1177/0890334418775624
4. Ghaheri, B. A., Lincoln, D., Mai, T., & Mace, J. C. (2022). Objective Improvement After Frenotomy for Posterior Tongue-Tie: A Prospective

Randomized Trial. *Otolaryngology--head and neck surgery : official journal of American Academy of Otolaryngology-Head and Neck Surgery, 166*(5), 976–984. https://doi.org/10.1177/01945998211039784

5. Santa Maria, C., Aby, J., Truong, M. T., Thakur, Y., Rea, S., & Messner, A. (2017). The Superior Labial Frenulum in Newborns: What Is Normal?. *Global pediatric health, 4*, 2333794X17718896. https://doi.org/10.1177/2333794X17718896

6. Malchodi, L., Wagner, K., Susi, A., Gorman, G., & Hisle-Gorman, E. (2019). Early Acid Suppression Therapy Exposure and Fracture in Young Children. *Pediatrics, 144*(1), e20182625. https://doi.org/10.1542/peds.2018-2625

7. Siegel, S. (2016). Aerophagia Induced Reflux in Breastfeeding Infants With Ankyloglossia and Shortened Maxillary Labial Frenula (Tongue and Lip Tie). *International Journal Of Clinical Pediatrics*, 5(1), 6-8.

8. Slagter, K. W., Raghoebar, G. M., Hamming, I., Meijer, J., & Vissink, A. (2021). Effect of frenotomy on breastfeeding and reflux: results from the BRIEF prospective longitudinal cohort study. *Clinical oral investigations, 25*(6), 3431–3439. https://doi.org/10.1007/s00784-020-03665-y

9. Hand, P., Olivi, G., Lajolo, C., Gioco, G., Marigo, L., Castagnola, R., & Cordaro, M. (2020). Short lingual frenum in infants, children and adolescents. Part 1: Breastfeeding and gastroesophageal reflux disease improvement after tethered oral tissues release. *European journal of paediatric dentistry, 21*(4), 309–317. https://doi.org/10.23804/ejpd.2020.21.04.10

10. Nyoni, Danai & Ganesan, Kandasamy & Parrish, Jennifer. (2017). Tongue Tie-Is it Related to Gastrointestinal Problems?. British Journal of Oral and Maxillofacial Surgery. 55. e157-e158. 10.1016/j.bjoms.2017.08.208.

11. Huang YS, Quo S, Berkowski JA, Guilleminault C (2015) Short Lingual Frenulum and Obstructive Sleep Apnea in Children. Int J Pediatr Res 1:003

12. Guilleminault, C., Huseni, S., & Lo, L. (2016). A frequent phenotype for paediatric sleep apnoea: short lingual frenulum. *ERJ open research, 2*(3), 00043-2016. https://doi.org/10.1183/23120541.00043-2016

13. Yoon, A. J., Zaghi, S., Ha, S., Law, C. S., Guilleminault, C., & Liu, S. Y. (2017). Ankyloglossia as a risk factor for maxillary hypoplasia and soft palate elongation: A functional - morphological study. *Orthodontics & craniofacial research, 20*(4), 237–244. https://doi.org/10.1111/ocr.12206

14. Villa, M. P., Evangelisti, M., Barreto, M., Cecili, M., & Kaditis, A. (2020). Short lingual frenulum as a risk factor for sleep-disordered breathing in school-age children. *Sleep medicine, 66*, 119–122. https://doi.org/10.1016/j.sleep.2019.09.019

15. Brożek-Mądry, E., Burska, Z., Steć, Z., Burghard, M., & Krzeski, A. (2021). Short lingual frenulum and head-forward posture in children with the risk of obstructive sleep apnea. *International journal of pediatric otorhinolaryngology, 144*, 110699. https://doi.org/10.1016/j.ijporl.2021.110699

16. Bussi, M. T., Corrêa, C. C., Cassettari, A. J., Giacomin, L. T., Faria, A. C., Moreira, A., Magalhães, I., Cunha, M., Weber, S., Zancanella, E., & Machado Júnior, A. J. (2021). Is ankyloglossia associated with obstructive sleep

apnea?. *Brazilian journal of otorhinolaryngology*, S1808-8694(21)00181-6. Advance online publication. https://doi.org/10.1016/j.bjorl.2021.09.008

17. Yuen, H. M., Au, C. T., Chu, W., Li, A. M., & Chan, K. C. (2022). Reduced tongue mobility: an unrecognized risk factor of childhood obstructive sleep apnea. *Sleep, 45*(1), zsab217. https://doi.org/10.1093/sleep/zsab217

18. Burska, Z., Burghard, M., Brożek-Mądry, E., Sierdziński, J., & Krzeski, A. (2022). Oral cavity morphology among children at risk of sleep disordered breathing. *European archives of paediatric dentistry : official journal of the European Academy of Paediatric Dentistry, 23*(3), 429–435. https://doi.org/10.1007/s40368-022-00701-1

19. Camacho, M., Certal, V., Abdullatif, J., Zaghi, S., Ruoff, C. M., Capasso, R., & Kushida, C. A. (2015). Myofunctional Therapy to Treat Obstructive Sleep Apnea: A Systematic Review and Meta-analysis. *Sleep, 38*(5), 669–675. https://doi.org/10.5665/sleep.4652

20. Zaghi, S., Valcu-Pinkerton, S., Jabara, M., Norouz-Knutsen, L., Govardhan, C., Moeller, J., Sinkus, V., Thorsen, R. S., Downing, V., Camacho, M., Yoon, A., Hang, W. M., Hockel, B., Guilleminault, C., & Liu, S. Y. (2019). Lingual frenuloplasty with myofunctional therapy: Exploring safety and efficacy in 348 cases. *Laryngoscope investigative otolaryngology, 4*(5), 489–496. https://doi.org/10.1002/lio2.297

Chapter 6: Small Jaws and Crooked Teeth

1. Mew M. (2014). Craniofacial dystrophy. A possible syndrome?. *British dental journal, 216*(10), 555–558. https://doi.org/10.1038/sj.bdj.2014.401

2. Grippaudo, Cristina, Patricia Valerio, Cristiana Romeo, Fabiana Fiasca, and Vincenzo Quinzi. 2020. "Bite and Sight: Is There a Correlation? Clinical Association between Dental Malocclusion and Visual Disturbances in Pediatric Patients" *Applied Sciences* 10, no. 17: 5913. https://doi.org/10.3390/app10175913

3. Ovsenik M. (2009). Incorrect orofacial functions until 5 years of age and their association with posterior crossbite. *American journal of orthodontics and dentofacial orthopedics : official publication of the American Association of Orthodontists, its constituent societies, and the American Board of Orthodontics, 136*(3), 375–381. https://doi.org/10.1016/j.ajodo.2008.03.018

4. Thilander, B., & Bjerklin, K. (2012). Posterior crossbite and temporomandibular disorders (TMDs): need for orthodontic treatment?. *European journal of orthodontics, 34*(6), 667–673. https://doi.org/10.1093/ejo/cjr095

5. Calvo-Henríquez, C., Neves, S. M., Branco, A. M., Lechien, J. R., Reinoso, F. B., Rojas, X. M., O'Connor-Reina, C., González-Guijarro, I., & Martínez Capoccioni, G. (2021). Relationship between short lingual frenulum and malocclusion. A multicentre study. *Acta otorrinolaringologica espanola*, S0001-6519(21)00031-5. Advance online publication. https://doi.org/10.1016/j.otorri.2021.01.002

6. Nunes, W. R., Jr, & Di Francesco, R. C. (2010). Variation of patterns of malocclusion by site of pharyngeal obstruction in children. *Archives of*

otolaryngology--head & neck surgery, *136*(11), 1116–1120. https://doi.org/10.1001/archoto.2010.187

7. Sonnesen, L., & Svensson, P. (2008). Temporomandibular disorders and psychological status in adult patients with a deep bite. *European journal of orthodontics*, *30*(6), 621–629. https://doi.org/10.1093/ejo/cjn044

8. McNarama, J.A.,(1981) Components of Class II Malocclusion in Children 8–10 Years of Age. *Angle Orthod* 51 (3): 177–202. https://doi.org/10.1043/0003-3219(1981)051<0177:COCIMI>2.0.CO;2

9. Guilleminault, C., Abad, V. C., Chiu, H. Y., Peters, B., & Quo, S. (2016). Missing teeth and pediatric obstructive sleep apnea. *Sleep & breathing = Schlaf & Atmung*, *20*(2), 561–568. https://doi.org/10.1007/s11325-015-1238-3

Chapter 7: Sleep and Airway Screenings

1. Marcus, C. L., Brooks, L. J., Draper, K. A., Gozal, D., Halbower, A. C., Jones, J., Schechter, M. S., Sheldon, S. H., Spruyt, K., Ward, S. D., Lehmann, C., Shiffman, R. N., & American Academy of Pediatrics (2012). Diagnosis and management of childhood obstructive sleep apnea syndrome. *Pediatrics*, *130*(3), 576–584. https://doi.org/10.1542/peds.2012-1671

2. Blunden, S., Lushington, K., Lorenzen, B., Ooi, T., Fung, F., & Kennedy, D. (2004). Are sleep problems under-recognised in general practice?. *Archives of disease in childhood*, *89*(8), 708–712. https://doi.org/10.1136/adc.2003.027011

3. Mindell, J. A., Bartle, A., Wahab, N. A., Ahn, Y., Ramamurthy, M. B., Huong, H. T., Kohyama, J., Ruangdaraganon, N., Sekartini, R., Teng, A., & Goh, D. Y. (2011). Sleep education in medical school curriculum: a glimpse across countries. *Sleep medicine*, *12*(9), 928–931. https://doi.org/10.1016/j.sleep.2011.07.001

4. American Dental Association, "The Role of Dentistry in the Treatment of Sleep Related Breathing Disorder." Accessed July 10, 2022. https://www.ada.org/-/media/project/ada-organization/ada/ada-org/files/resources/research/the-role-of-dentistry-in-sleep-related-breathing-disorders.pdf

5. Stark, T. R., Pozo-Alonso, M., Daniels, R., & Camacho, M. (2018). Pediatric Considerations for Dental Sleep Medicine. *Sleep medicine clinics*, *13*(4), 531–548. https://doi.org/10.1016/j.jsmc.2018.08.002

6. Luzzi, V., Ierardo, G., Di Carlo, G., Saccucci, M., & Polimeni, A. (2019). Obstructive sleep apnea syndrome in the pediatric age: the role of the dentist. *European review for medical and pharmacological sciences*, *23*(1 Suppl), 9–14. https://doi.org/10.26355/eurrev_201903_17341

7. Giuca, M. R., Carli, E., Lardani, L., Pasini, M., Miceli, M., & Fambrini, E. (2021). Pediatric Obstructive Sleep Apnea Syndrome: Emerging Evidence and Treatment Approach. *TheScientificWorldJournal*, *2021*, 5591251. https://doi.org/10.1155/2021/5591251

8. Moin Anwer, H. M., Albagieh, H. N., Kalladka, M., Chiang, H. K., Malik, S., McLaren, S. W., & Khan, J. (2021). The role of the dentist in the diagnosis and management of pediatric obstructive sleep apnea. *The Saudi dental journal*, *33*(7), 424–433. https://doi.org/10.1016/j.sdentj.2021.02.001

9. Oh, J. S., Zaghi, S., Peterson, C., Law, C. S., Silva, D., & Yoon, A. J. (2021). Determinants of Sleep-Disordered Breathing During the Mixed Dentition: Development of a Functional Airway Evaluation Screening Tool (FAIREST-6). *Pediatric dentistry*, *43*(4), 262–272.
10. Calvo-Henriquez, C., Martins-Neves, S., Martinez-Capoccioni, G., Neves-Leal, D., Ruano-Ravina, A., Faraldo-García, A., Lowy-Benoliel, A., & Martin-Martin, C. (2019). Validation of the Vertical Facial Growth Screening Test. *Clinical pediatrics*, *58*(11-12), 1187–1193. https://doi.org/10.1177/0009922819868684
11. Ikävalko, T., Närhi, M., Eloranta, A. M., Lintu, N., Myllykangas, R., Vierola, A., Tuomilehto, H., Lakka, T., & Pahkala, R. (2018). Predictors of sleep disordered breathing in children: the PANIC study. *European journal of orthodontics*, *40*(3), 268–272. https://doi.org/10.1093/ejo/cjx056
12. Weiss, T. M., Atanasov, S., & Calhoun, K. H. (2005). The association of tongue scalloping with obstructive sleep apnea and related sleep pathology. *Otolaryngology--head and neck surgery : official journal of American Academy of Otolaryngology-Head and Neck Surgery*, *133*(6), 966–971. https://doi.org/10.1016/j.otohns.2005.07.018
13. Oh, J. S., Zaghi, S., Ghodousi, N., Peterson, C., Silva, D., Lavigne, G. J., & Yoon, A. J. (2021). Determinants of probable sleep bruxism in a pediatric mixed dentition population: a multivariate analysis of mouth vs. nasal breathing, tongue mobility, and tonsil size. *Sleep medicine*, *77*, 7–13. https://doi.org/10.1016/j.sleep.2020.11.007
14. Manfredini, D., Guarda-Nardini, L., Marchese-Ragona, R., & Lobbezoo, F. (2015). Theories on possible temporal relationships between sleep bruxism and obstructive sleep apnea events. An expert opinion. *Sleep & breathing = Schlaf & Atmung*, *19*(4), 1459–1465. https://doi.org/10.1007/s11325-015-1163-5
15. Balasubramaniam, R., Klasser, G. D., Cistulli, P. A., & Lavigne, G. J. (2014). The link between sleep bruxism, sleep disordered breathing and temporomandibular disorders: an evidence-based review. *J Dent Sleep Med*, *1*(1), 27-37.
16. Lavigne, G. J., Khoury, S., Abe, S., Yamaguchi, T., & Raphael, K. (2008). Bruxism physiology and pathology: an overview for clinicians. *Journal of oral rehabilitation*, *35*(7), 476–494. https://doi.org/10.1111/j.1365-2842.2008.01881.x
17. Oh, J. S., Zaghi, S., Ghodousi, N., Peterson, C., Silva, D., Lavigne, G. J., & Yoon, A. J. (2021). Determinants of probable sleep bruxism in a pediatric mixed dentition population: a multivariate analysis of mouth vs. nasal breathing, tongue mobility, and tonsil size. *Sleep medicine*, *77*, 7–13. https://doi.org/10.1016/j.sleep.2020.11.007
18. DiFrancesco, R. C., Junqueira, P. A., Trezza, P. M., de Faria, M. E., Frizzarini, R., & Zerati, F. E. (2004). Improvement of bruxism after T & A surgery. *International journal of pediatric otorhinolaryngology*, *68*(4), 441–445. https://doi.org/10.1016/j.ijporl.2003.11.022
19. Eftekharian, A., Raad, N., & Gholami-Ghasri, N. (2008). Bruxism and adenotonsillectomy. *International journal of pediatric otorhinolaryngology*, *72*(4), 509–511. https://doi.org/10.1016/j.ijporl.2008.01.006

20. Rouse, J.S. (2010). The Bruxism Triad Sleep bruxism , sleep disturbance , and sleep-related GERD.
21. Guilleminault, C., Abad, V. C., Chiu, H. Y., Peters, B., & Quo, S. (2016). Missing teeth and pediatric obstructive sleep apnea. *Sleep & breathing = Schlaf & Atmung, 20*(2), 561–568. https://doi.org/10.1007/s11325-015-1238-3
22. Chervin, R. D., Hedger, K., Dillon, J. E., & Pituch, K. J. (2000). Pediatric sleep questionnaire (PSQ): validity and reliability of scales for sleep-disordered breathing, snoring, sleepiness, and behavioral problems. *Sleep medicine, 1*(1), 21–32. https://doi.org/10.1016/s1389-9457(99)00009-x
23. Lin, C. H., & Guilleminault, C. (2011). Current hypopnea scoring criteria underscore pediatric sleep disordered breathing. *Sleep medicine, 12*(7), 720–729. https://doi.org/10.1016/j.sleep.2011.04.004
24. Bariani, R., Guimarães, T. M., Cappellette, M., Junior, Moreira, G., & Fujita, R. R. (2020). The impact of positive airway pressure on midface growth: a literature review. *Brazilian journal of otorhinolaryngology, 86*(5), 647–653. https://doi.org/10.1016/j.bjorl.2020.05.010

Chapter 8: Adenoids, Tonsils and Grommets

1. Mitchell, R. B., Archer, S. M., Ishman, S. L., Rosenfeld, R. M., Coles, S., Finestone, S. A., Friedman, N. R., Giordano, T., Hildrew, D. M., Kim, T. W., Lloyd, R. M., Parikh, S. R., Shulman, S. T., Walner, D. L., Walsh, S. A., & Nnacheta, L. C. (2019). Clinical Practice Guideline: Tonsillectomy in Children (Update). *Otolaryngology--head and neck surgery : official journal of American Academy of Otolaryngology-Head and Neck Surgery, 160*(1_suppl), S1–S42. https://doi.org/10.1177/0194599818801757
2. Erickson, B. K., Larson, D. R., St Sauver, J. L., Meverden, R. A., & Orvidas, L. J. (2009). Changes in incidence and indications of tonsillectomy and adenotonsillectomy, 1970-2005. *Otolaryngology--head and neck surgery : official journal of American Academy of Otolaryngology-Head and Neck Surgery, 140*(6), 894–901. https://doi.org/10.1016/j.otohns.2009.01.044
3. Bhattacharjee, R., Kheirandish-Gozal, L., Spruyt, K., Mitchell, R. B., Promchiarak, J., Simakajornboon, N., Kaditis, A. G., Splaingard, D., Splaingard, M., Brooks, L. J., Marcus, C. L., Sin, S., Arens, R., Verhulst, S. L., & Gozal, D. (2010). Adenotonsillectomy outcomes in treatment of obstructive sleep apnea in children: a multicenter retrospective study. *American journal of respiratory and critical care medicine, 182*(5), 676–683. https://doi.org/10.1164/rccm.200912-1930OC
4. Stupak, H. D., & Park, S. Y. (2018). Gravitational forces, negative pressure and facial structure in the genesis of airway dysfunction during sleep: a review of the paradigm. *Sleep medicine, 51*, 125–132. https://doi.org/10.1016/j.sleep.2018.06.016
5. Stupak, H., 2020. *Rethinking Rhinoplasty and Facial Surgery*. Springer Nature Switzerland.
6. Yoon, A., Abdelwahab, M., Bockow, R., Vakili, A., Lovell, K., Chang, I., Ganguly, R., Liu, S. Y., Kushida, C., & Hong, C. (2022). Impact of rapid palatal

expansion on the size of adenoids and tonsils in children. *Sleep medicine*, *92*, 96–102. https://doi.org/10.1016/j.sleep.2022.02.011

7. Dm, Christian Guilleminault, C Guilleminault and Shannon S. Sullivan. "Towards Restoration of Continuous Nasal Breathing as the Ultimate Treatment Goal in Pediatric Obstructive Sleep Apnea." (2014).

8. Gray L. P. (1975). Results of 310 cases of rapid maxillary expansion selected for medical reasons. *The Journal of laryngology and otology*, *89*(6), 601–614. https://doi.org/10.1017/s0022215100080804

9. Kim, S. J., Donovan, D. M., Blanchard, S. B., Kowolik, J. E., & Eckert, G. J. (2008). The relationship between acute otitis media and the anatomic form of the hard palate. *Pediatric dentistry*, *30*(1), 9–14.

10. Fagundes, N., Rabello, N. M., Maia, L. C., Normando, D., & Mello, K. (2017). Can rapid maxillary expansion cause auditory improvement in children and adolescents with hearing loss? A systematic review. *The Angle orthodontist*, *87*(6), 886–896. https://doi.org/10.2319/021517-111.1

11. Kılıç, N., Yörük, Ö., Kılıç, S. C., Çatal, G., & Kurt, S. (2016). Rapid maxillary expansion versus middle ear tube placement: Comparison of hearing improvements in children with resistance otitis media with effusion. *The Angle orthodontist*, *86*(5), 761–767. https://doi.org/10.2319/101515-693.1

12. Kılıç, N., Yörük, Ö., & Kılıç, S. C. (2021). An alternative treatment approach for patients with resistant otitis media with effusion and dysfunctional Eustachian tube. *The Angle orthodontist*, *91*(6), 772–777. https://doi.org/10.2319/021421-127.1

Chapter 9: Palate Expansion

1. Gray L. P. (1975). Results of 310 cases of rapid maxillary expansion selected for medical reasons. *The Journal of laryngology and otology*, *89*(6), 601–614. https://doi.org/10.1017/s0022215100080804

2. Calvo-Henriquez, C., Capasso, R., Chiesa-Estomba, C., Liu, S. Y., Martins-Neves, S., Castedo, E., O'Connor-Reina, C., Ruano-Ravina, A., & Kahn, S. (2020). The role of pediatric maxillary expansion on nasal breathing. A systematic review and metanalysis. International journal of pediatric otorhinolaryngology, 135, 110139. https://doi.org/10.1016/j.ijporl.2020.110139

3. Machado-Júnior, A. J., Zancanella, E., & Crespo, A. N. (2016). Rapid maxillary expansion and obstructive sleep apnea: A review and meta-analysis. *Medicina oral, patologia oral y cirugia bucal*, *21*(4), e465–e469. https://doi.org/10.4317/medoral.21073

4. Camacho, M., Chang, E. T., Song, S. A., Abdullatif, J., Zaghi, S., Pirelli, P., Certal, V., & Guilleminault, C. (2017). Rapid maxillary expansion for pediatric obstructive sleep apnea: A systematic review and meta-analysis. *The Laryngoscope*, *127*(7), 1712–1719. https://doi.org/10.1002/lary.26352

5. Iwasaki, T., Saitoh, I., Takemoto, Y., Inada, E., Kakuno, E., Kanomi, R., Hayasaki, H., & Yamasaki, Y. (2013). Tongue posture improvement and pharyngeal airway enlargement as secondary effects of rapid maxillary expansion: a cone-beam computed tomography study. *American journal of*

orthodontics and dentofacial orthopedics : official publication of the American Association of Orthodontists, its constituent societies, and the American Board of Orthodontics, 143(2), 235–245. https://doi.org/10.1016/j.ajodo.2012.09.014

6. Zaffanello, M., Piacentini, G., Lippi, G., Fanos, V., Gasperi, E., & Nosetti, L. (2017). Obstructive sleep-disordered breathing, enuresis and combined disorders in children: chance or related association?. *Swiss medical weekly, 147*, w14400. https://doi.org/10.4414/smw.2017.14400

7. Shafiek, H., Evangelisti, M., Abd-Elwahab, N. H., Barreto, M., Villa, M. P., & Mahmoud, M. I. (2020). Obstructive Sleep Apnea in School-Aged Children Presented with Nocturnal Enuresis. *Lung, 198*(1), 187–194. https://doi.org/10.1007/s00408-019-00304-6

8. Khalaf, K., Mansour, D., Sawalha, Z., & Habrawi, S. (2021). Rapid Maxillary Expansion and Nocturnal Enuresis in Children and Adolescents: A Systematic Review of Controlled Clinical Trials. TheScientificWorldJournal, 2021, 1004629. https://doi.org/10.1155/2021/1004629

9. de Medeiros Alves, A. C., de Medeiros Padilha, H., de Andrade Barbalho, A. L., Gonçalves Tomaz, A. F., Gomes Pereira, H. S., & Rabelo Caldas, S. (2021). Influence of rapid maxillary expansion on nocturnal enuresis in children. *The Angle orthodontist, 91*(5), 680–691. https://doi.org/10.2319/042520-355.1

10. Cohen, SA., Malocclusion and Its Far Reach Effects. *JAMA.* 1922;79(23):1895–1897. doi:10.1001/jama.1922.02640230005002

Chapter 10: Myofunctional Therapy

1. Camacho, M., Certal, V., Abdullatif, J., Zaghi, S., Ruoff, C. M., Capasso, R., & Kushida, C. A. (2015). Myofunctional Therapy to Treat Obstructive Sleep Apnea: A Systematic Review and Meta-analysis. *Sleep, 38*(5), 669–675. https://doi.org/10.5665/sleep.4652

2. Carrasco-Llatas, M., O'Connor-Reina, C., & Calvo-Henríquez, C. (2021). The Role of Myofunctional Therapy in Treating Sleep-Disordered Breathing: A State-of-the-Art Review. *International journal of environmental research and public health, 18*(14), 7291. https://doi.org/10.3390/ijerph18147291

3. Bandyopadhyay, A., Kaneshiro, K., & Camacho, M. (2020). Effect of myofunctional therapy on children with obstructive sleep apnea: a meta-analysis. *Sleep medicine, 75*, 210–217. https://doi.org/10.1016/j.sleep.2020.08.003

4. de Felício, C. M., da Silva Dias, F. V., & Trawitzki, L. (2018). Obstructive sleep apnea: focus on myofunctional therapy. *Nature and science of sleep, 10*, 271–286. https://doi.org/10.2147/NSS.S141132

5. Huang, Y. S., & Guilleminault, C. (2017). Pediatric Obstructive Sleep Apnea: Where Do We Stand?. *Advances in oto-rhino-laryngology, 80*, 136–144. https://doi.org/10.1159/000470885

6. Villa, M. P., Evangelisti, M., Martella, S., Barreto, M., & Del Pozzo, M. (2017). Can myofunctional therapy increase tongue tone and reduce symptoms in children with sleep-disordered breathing?. *Sleep & breathing = Schlaf & Atmung, 21*(4), 1025–1032. https://doi.org/10.1007/s11325-017-1489-2

7. Lee, S. Y., Guilleminault, C., Chiu, H. Y., & Sullivan, S. S. (2015). Mouth breathing, "nasal disuse," and pediatric sleep-disordered breathing. *Sleep & breathing = Schlaf & Atmung*, *19*(4), 1257–1264. https://doi.org/10.1007/s11325-015-1154-6
8. Levrini, L., Lorusso, P., Caprioglio, A., Magnani, A., Diaféria, G., Bittencourt, L., & Bommarito, S. (2014). Model of oronasal rehabilitation in children with obstructive sleep apnea syndrome undergoing rapid maxillary expansion: Research review. *Sleep science (Sao Paulo, Brazil)*, *7*(4), 225–233. https://doi.org/10.1016/j.slsci.2014.11.002
9. Moeller, Joy & Paskay, Licia & Gelb, Michael. (2014). Myofunctional Therapy : A Novel Treatment of Pediatric Sleep-Disordered Breathing. Sleep Medicine Clinics. 9. 235–243. 10.1016/j.jsmc.2014.03.002.
10. Guilleminault, C., Huang, Y. S., Monteyrol, P. J., Sato, R., Quo, S., & Lin, C. H. (2013). Critical role of myofascial reeducation in pediatric sleep-disordered breathing. *Sleep medicine*, *14*(6), 518–525. https://doi.org/10.1016/j.sleep.2013.01.013
11. Gozal, D., Ismail, M., & Brockmann, P. E. (2021). Alternatives to surgery in children with mild OSA. *World journal of otorhinolaryngology - head and neck surgery*, *7*(3), 228–235. https://doi.org/10.1016/j.wjorl.2021.03.005

Chapter 11: Airway Health in Adulthood

1. Lamberg, S. *Sleep-related breathing disorders can impact pregnancy*. Dental Sleep Practice - Sleep Apnea Publication & Online CE. Retrieved July 11, 2022, from https://dentalsleeppractice.com/ce-articles/sleep-related-breathing-disorders-during-pregnancy-the-impact-of-intervention-on-maternal-and-fetal-health-outcomes/
2. Park, Steven Y. 2012. *Sleep, Interrupted: A Physician Reveals the #1 Reason Why so Many of Us Are Sick and Tired*. New York: Jodev Press.
3. Palombini L, Lopes M, Tufik S, Christian G, Bittencourt LRA. Upper airway resistance syndrome: still not recognized and not treated. Sleep Sci.2011;4(2):72-78
4. Amdo, T., Hasaneen, N., Gold, M. S., & Gold, A. R. (2016). Somatic syndromes, insomnia, anxiety, and stress among sleep disordered breathing patients. *Sleep & breathing = Schlaf & Atmung*, *20*(2), 759–768. https://doi.org/10.1007/s11325-015-1296-6
5. Broderick, J. E., Gold, M. S., Amin, M. M., & Gold, A. R. (2014). The association of somatic arousal with the symptoms of upper airway resistance syndrome. *Sleep medicine*, *15*(4), 436–443. https://doi.org/10.1016/j.sleep.2014.01.014
6. Gold A. R. (2011). Functional somatic syndromes, anxiety disorders and the upper airway: a matter of paradigms. *Sleep medicine reviews*, *15*(6), 389–401. https://doi.org/10.1016/j.smrv.2010.11.004
7. Gold, A. R., Dipalo, F., Gold, M. S., & Broderick, J. (2004). Inspiratory airflow dynamics during sleep in women with fibromyalgia. *Sleep*, *27*(3), 459–466. https://doi.org/10.1093/sleep/27.3.459

8. Gold, A. R., Dipalo, F., Gold, M. S., & O'Hearn, D. (2003). The symptoms and signs of upper airway resistance syndrome: a link to the functional somatic syndromes. *Chest, 123*(1), 87–95. https://doi.org/10.1378/chest.123.1.87

9. Gold, M. S., Amdo, T., Hasaneen, N., & Gold, A. R. (2016). Somatic arousal and sleepiness/fatigue among patients with sleep-disordered breathing. *Sleep & breathing = Schlaf & Atmung, 20*(2), 749–758. https://doi.org/10.1007/s11325-015-1294-8

10. Proothi, M., Grazina, V., & Gold, A. R. (2019). Chronic insomnia remitting after maxillomandibular advancement for mild obstructive sleep apnea: a case series. *Journal of medical case reports, 13*(1), 252. https://doi.org/10.1186/s13256-019-2182-9

11. Huffington Post. "Nocturnal Teeth Grinding May Suggest a Sleep Disorder." Accessed 11 Jul 2021. https://www.huffpost.com/entry/teeth-grinding-sleep_b_4124494

12. Manfredini, D., Guarda-Nardini, L., Marchese-Ragona, R., & Lobbezoo, F. (2015). Theories on possible temporal relationships between sleep bruxism and obstructive sleep apnea events. An expert opinion. *Sleep & breathing = Schlaf & Atmung, 19*(4), 1459–1465. https://doi.org/10.1007/s11325-015-1163-5

13. Balasubramaniam, R., Klasser, G. D., Cistulli, P. A., & Lavigne, G. J. (2014). The link between sleep bruxism, sleep disordered breathing and temporomandibular disorders: an evidence-based review. *J Dent Sleep Med, 1*(1), 27-37.

14. Singh, N. (2011) Sleep Bruxism Related Tooth Wear as a Clinical Marker of Obstructive Sleep Apnea/Hypopnea Syndrome in Children. (Doctoral dissertation, Tufts University). Tufts Digital Library. http://hdl.handle.net/10427/011090

15. Gagnon, Y., Mayer, P., Morisson, F., Rompré, P. H., & Lavigne, G. J. (2004). Aggravation of respiratory disturbances by the use of an occlusal splint in apneic patients: a pilot study. *The International journal of prosthodontics, 17*(4), 447–453.

16. American College of Prosthodontics. "ACP Position Statement - Role of Oral Devices in Managing Sleep-disordered Breathing Patient." Accessed 11 July 2022. https://www.prosthodontics.org/assets/1/7/16.Role_of_Oral_Devices_in_Managing_Sleep-disordered_Breathing_Patients.pdf

17. Peppard, P. E., Young, T., Palta, M., Dempsey, J., & Skatrud, J. (2000). Longitudinal study of moderate weight change and sleep-disordered breathing. *JAMA, 284*(23), 3015–3021. https://doi.org/10.1001/jama.284.23.3015

18. Phillips, C. L., Grunstein, R. R., Darendeliler, M. A., Mihailidou, A. S., Srinivasan, V. K., Yee, B. J., Marks, G. B., & Cistulli, P. A. (2013). Health outcomes of continuous positive airway pressure versus oral appliance treatment for obstructive sleep apnea: a randomized controlled trial. *American journal of respiratory and critical care medicine, 187*(8), 879–887. https://doi.org/10.1164/rccm.201212-2223OC

19. Lan, M. C., Liu, S. Y., Lan, M. Y., Modi, R., & Capasso, R. (2015). Lateral pharyngeal wall collapse associated with hypoxemia in obstructive sleep

apnea. *The Laryngoscope*, *125*(10), 2408–2412. https://doi.org/10.1002/lary.25126

20. Boyd, S. B., Chigurupati, R., Cillo, J. E., Jr, Eskes, G., Goodday, R., Meisami, T., Viozzi, C. F., Waite, P., & Wilson, J. (2019). Maxillomandibular Advancement Improves Multiple Health-Related and Functional Outcomes in Patients With Obstructive Sleep Apnea: A Multicenter Study. *Journal of oral and maxillofacial surgery : official journal of the American Association of Oral and Maxillofacial Surgeons*, *77*(2), 352–370. https://doi.org/10.1016/j.joms.2018.06.173

21. Lin, C. H., Chin, W. C., Huang, Y. S., Wang, P. F., Li, K. K., Pirelli, P., Chen, Y. H., & Guilleminault, C. (2020). Objective and subjective long term outcome of maxillomandibular advancement in obstructive sleep apnea. *Sleep medicine*, *74*, 289–296. https://doi.org/10.1016/j.sleep.2020.05.024

22. Liu, S. Y., Awad, M., Riley, R., & Capasso, R. (2019). The Role of the Revised Stanford Protocol in Today's Precision Medicine. *Sleep medicine clinics*, *14*(1), 99–107. https://doi.org/10.1016/j.jsmc.2018.10.013

23. Liu, S. Y., Wayne Riley, R., Pogrel, A., & Guilleminault, C. (2019). Sleep Surgery in the Era of Precision Medicine. *Atlas of the oral and maxillofacial surgery clinics of North America*, *27*(1), 1–5. https://doi.org/10.1016/j.cxom.2018.11.012

24. Liu, S. Y., Riley, R. W., & Yu, M. S. (2020). Surgical Algorithm for Obstructive Sleep Apnea: An Update. *Clinical and experimental otorhinolaryngology*, *13*(3), 215–224. https://doi.org/10.21053/ceo.2020.01053

25. Williams, R., Patel, V., Chen, Y. F., Tangbumrungtham, N., Thamboo, A., Most, S. P., Nayak, J. V., & Liu, S. (2019). The Upper Airway Nasal Complex: Structural Contribution to Persistent Nasal Obstruction. *Otolaryngology--head and neck surgery : official journal of American Academy of Otolaryngology-Head and Neck Surgery*, *161*(1), 171–177. https://doi.org/10.1177/0194599819838262

26. Yoon, A., Guilleminault, C., Zaghi, S., & Liu, S. Y. (2020). Distraction Osteogenesis Maxillary Expansion (DOME) for adult obstructive sleep apnea patients with narrow maxilla and nasal floor. *Sleep medicine*, *65*, 172–176. https://doi.org/10.1016/j.sleep.2019.06.002

27. Iwasaki, T., Yoon, A., Guilleminault, C., Yamasaki, Y., & Liu, S. Y. (2020). How does distraction osteogenesis maxillary expansion (DOME) reduce severity of obstructive sleep apnea?. *Sleep & breathing = Schlaf & Atmung*, *24*(1), 287–296. https://doi.org/10.1007/s11325-019-01948-7

28. Liu, S. Y., Yoon, A., Abdelwahab, M., & Yu, M. S. (2022). Feasibility of distraction osteogenesis maxillary expansion in patients with persistent nasal obstruction after septoplasty. *International forum of allergy & rhinology*, *12*(6), 868–871. https://doi.org/10.1002/alr.22931

29. Thuler, E., Rabelo, F., Yui, M., Tominaga, Q., Dos Santos, V., Jr, & Arap, S. S. (2021). Correlation between the transverse dimension of the maxilla, upper airway obstructive site, and OSA severity. *Journal of clinical sleep medicine : JCSM : official publication of the American Academy of Sleep Medicine*, *17*(7), 1465–1473. https://doi.org/10.5664/jcsm.9226

ABOUT THE AUTHOR

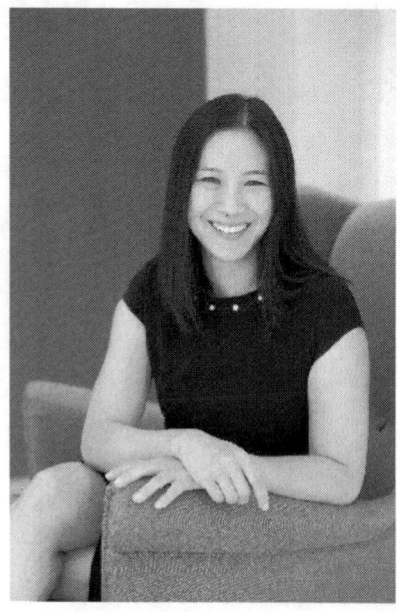

Dr. Lim was one of Australia's first handful of dentists to obtain a qualification in dental sleep medicine.

She has been involved in managing snoring and obstructive sleep apnoea for over a decade and has seen the physical, developmental, mental, and emotional problems that are often associated with these breathing disturbances throughout the lifespan.

Her mission is to highlight root causes and promote airway health, or a shift from managing disease and symptoms towards ensuring healthy nasal breathing and good airway development from infancy.

She works in private practice and has a special focus on unlocking greater health and wellness through addressing tongue ties, oral dysfunction (during infant feeding, swallowing, breathing, chewing, and speech), and guiding good jaw development during childhood.

To find out more, visit
DrShereenLim.com.au

Made in United States
Orlando, FL
19 October 2024

52871161R00109